Dedicated to my nephew, David Gimelfarb,

Lost in Costa Rico in 2009

Order this book online at www.trafford.com
or email orders@trafford.com

Most Trafford titles are also available at major online book retailers.

© Copyright 2011 Chester Litvin, PhD.

All rights reserved. No part of this publication may be reproduced, stored in a retrieval system, or transmitted, in any form or by any means, electronic, mechanical, photocopying, recording, or otherwise, without the written prior permission of the author.

Print information available on the last page.

ISBN: 978-1-4269-7336-9 (sc)

Library of Congress Control Number: 2011910669

Trafford rev. 05/07/2015

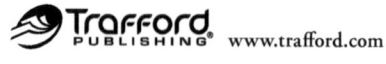 www.trafford.com

North America & international
toll-free: 1 888 232 4444 (USA & Canada)
fax: 812 355 4082

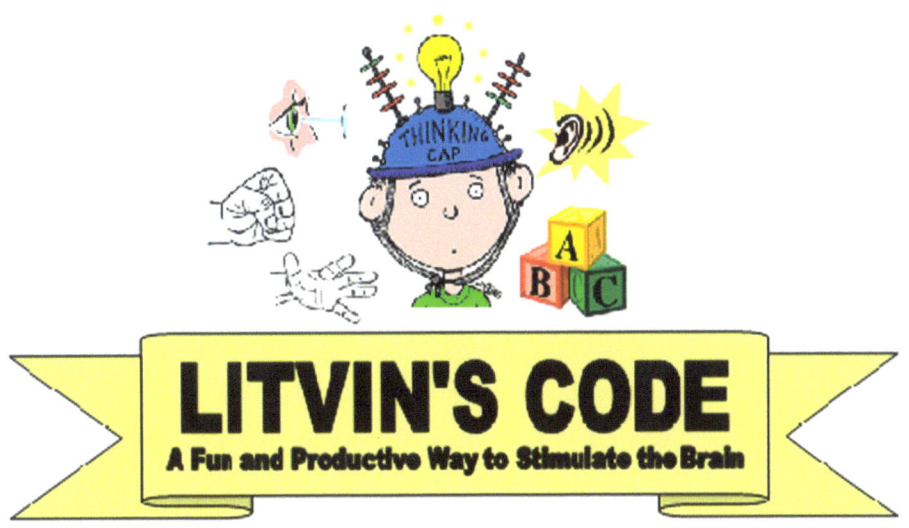

LITVIN'S CODE
A Fun and Productive Way to Stimulate the Brain

WRITTEN BY: Dr. Chester Litvin, Ph.D.
ILLUSTRATION BY: Dr. Niki Martirosyan, Ph.D.

Chester Litvin, Ph.D., Clinical Psychologist

How to increase learning - the psychological stimulation of the brain

by method of psychoconduction.

If you were called lazy or stupid and have problems with your memory, concentration, decision making, it can be because your brain is not stimulated enough to process complex information. We are using the new approach for non-invasive brain stimulation to wake up your sleeping brain. By using only the simple symbols we are significantly simplifying the identification of the information and capacity to manipulate it. The process of translating the same information to visual, audio, kinesthetic, tactile, olfactory and etc. modes of expression we call psychoconduction. In this book we explore the concept of positions, as part of binary arithmetic, and translation of the symbol. The different forms, which contains the translated information called the Litvin's Code. In future publications we hope to explore the mathematic and grammar by using psychoconduction and Litvin's Code instead of recognition of numbers and letters by contours.

The task to keep information in most simple form is always a struggle. In our discovery we are not changing any information, but somehow we want to change the structure of the brain's cells to process information. It is not a problem anymore to have simple representation of information. The complex information can become simple and acceptable by simple brain cells. For new process of information we are substituting the complex cells by simple brain cells. Our goal is to change the way how the information is carried but is not changing the information itself. We are providing opportunities to use simple brain cells instead of damaged or not effective complex cells. The psychoconduction is the process of educating the simple cell to act as a complex. Our work was done with the brain cells but in future can be done with other body cells.

By translating the complex information to the simple form we are educating the simple brain cells. We can use the simple form to transmit the complex information. The goal is to stimulate the simple cells to increase learning. The stimulated brain can learn how to process information in more efficient way. In our work we enhance and make more effective the previous not sufficient ways of processing the information. We stimulate brain by various combinations of positions, which are empty or filled up with simple symbol.

The wide brain stimulation with simple symbols is an important part of learning. When we are disregarding the stimulation of different part of the brain, we are processing information through the visual stimuli and putting the big emphasis on the visual faculty. The educational contribution of psychoconduction is to widen opportunity of the brain stimulation. When we are using memory of entire brain, we are enhancing the learning, increasing the attention and concentration. By using psychoconduction we are translating visual, audio and kinesthetic stimuli between various modes of expression.

The psychoconduction is bringing the fun to the learning process. Some. have difficulty processing video information, but others are more impaired in processing of audio or kinesthetic. During the translation of information between different modes we are using the empty and full positions, and we are not changing any content of learning. We are using the same logical system for different perceptions. The result is very promising. The students, with problems in learning, from the very young to the old age, were learning to process information with the different levels of complexity. As a result, the youngsters, later in life did not drop out of the high school and all of them continued the education in the college. A student with severe dyslexia, despite all predictions, has not dropped from the school and completed her education in the university. The elderly people with dementia got increased recall of information.

The psychoconduction helped variety of students to increase their academic performance and increase attention, concentration, also ability to focus and to complete tasks. It provides the easy translation to visual, audio, kinesthetic mode, the automatic use of groups, combinations, and permutation and factorial representations. The binary sequence represented by empty and full positions and the content of the position depends on the sequenced number of position, filled up with symbol. The combination part of psychoconduction is the empty and filled up positions joint together and uniquely represents the numbers and the letters.

The content of empty position is always zero and does not change. In binary arithmetic the sequential numbers of position are starting with one with the increment by one for the next position and ext. It could be unlimited number of positions in the sequence. The content of the filled up position is a binary number, which depends on the sequential number of the position. The content of the first position starts with 1, then the next position twice bigger and has content equal to 2, then the next position is twice bigger and has content of four, and again the next position has content of eight and etc. To arrive to the needed number or letter we are adding contents only of filled up positions, because the empty position has value of zero.

The little children without any difficulties are memorizing the combination of empty and full position, which could be represented by the audio, video, kinesthetic, olfactory, music and tactile modes of expression. The best way for little children is to use kinesthetic or tactile representation of the positions, because the learning for them also is the fun. The brain is easily processing the patterns of simple symbol that in audio, visual kinesthetic and olfactory modes has the same meaning. By using psychoconduction the complex information which people with learning disabilities had difficult and sometimes were not able to process at all, became very simple.

The psychoconduction allows us:
- understand the notion of ascending direction and the quick recognition of information.
-understand the relationship between empty, and filled position and we are simplifying the process of addition, subtraction, division and multiplication.
- have logical connection between empty and filled up positions and to spell words and sentences.

When the brain is not performing adequately due to physiological limitation, the process of the recognition of the complex spatial information is very complicated and confusing. Intuitively, we can use approximation by contours. The approximation helps us to make a guess. The guess could be right or wrong. We need to recognize the tremendous effort of the brain to bring us to this point.

By using psychoconduction we make the process of recognition less painful and less time consuming. We don't look for matching of spatial image through complicated scanning. We are providing constant numerical reference by checking if the position is filled or empty. We are successfully training the brain to overcome weakness in the processing of information. The psychoconduction protects the brain against unnecessary stress of recognition and allows focusing on the process. We tune areas of the brain against the other areas to achieve the congruency in the responses.

In this book the psychoconduction utilizes the notion of positions as part of binary arithmetic, which is completely different from memorizing contours. When the symbol is in the different position then the meaning is changing. It allows the person to have a stable relationship with the simplest symbol, instead of complicated contours. We also are providing the mathematical references. The psychoconduction allows to process information through audio, visual, kinesthetic and tactile expressions.

.

Contents

INTRODUCTION

GREEN LESSONS 6
GREEN LESSONS, LESSON 1, Figure 1 7
COUNT NUMBER OF OBJECTS IN EACH PICTURE 26
BLUE LESSONS, Figure 1 – 8 27
BLUE LESSONS, Exercise, Figure 1 – 8 32
BLUE LESSONS, Figure 9 – 16 36
BLUE LESSONS, Exercise, Figure 9 – 16 42
BLUE LESSONS, Figure 17 – 24 46
BLUE LESSONS, Exercise, Figure 17 – 24 50
BLUE LESSONS, Figure 25 – 29 54
BLUE LESSONS, Exercise, Figure 25 – 29 56
BLUE LESSONS, Figure 30 – 31 59
BLUE LESSONS, Exercise, Figure 30 – 31 60
INTRODUCTION TO   POSITIONS 61
INTRODUCTION TO POSITIONS: LESSON 1 – 31 62
INTRODUCTION TO SIGNS 78
INTRODUCTION TO SIGNS: LESSON 1, Exercise 1 – 5 79
INTRODUCTION TO SIGNS: TRAINING, Exercise 1 – 3 82

Green

Lessons

GREEN LESSONS, LESSON 1, Figure 1

In Figure 1, the **_visual_** display has two pictures with boxes. The pictures have different audio representations and different visual displays. The audio representation of a knock represents a filled up position and a double knock represents an empty position. In the first picture we have two empty spaces and the audio representations are **double knock and double knock**. In the second picture, the first position is filled up with a symbol and the second position is empty.

The **_audio_** representation for the second picture consists of a **knock and double knock**.

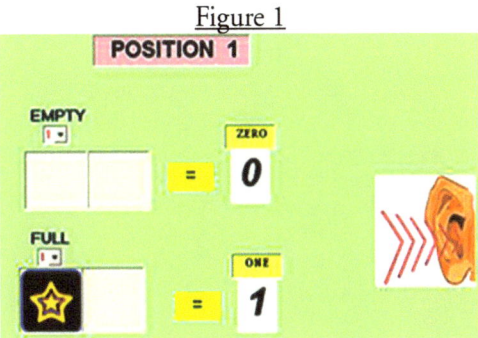

Figure 1

The **_kinesthetic_** representation of a filled up position is the clenching of the right hand. An empty position is represented by the clenching of the left hand. The kinesthetic representation for the first picture is the clenching of the left hand twice which is equal to the value of zero. The kinesthetic representation of the second picture is the clenching of the right hand, then the left hand. This signifies a mathematical value equal to one.

GREEN LESSONS, LESSON 1, Figure 2

In Figure 2, we have a **_visual_** display of two pictures with boxes. Both pictures have the same audio representations. The figures have different symbols in the filled positions. In the first picture the symbol is a star and in the second picture, a red ball. The shape of the symbols does not change the mathematical meaning and the pictures correspond to the same audio signals. In both pictures the first position is filled with a symbol and the second position is empty.

The **_audio_** representation for both pictures consists of a **knock and double knock**, where a knock represents a filled up position and a double knock represents an empty position.

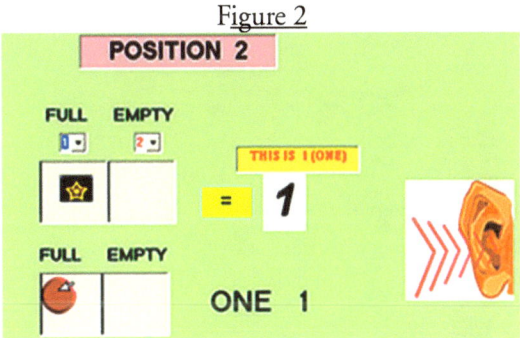

Figure 2

The **_kinesthetic_** representation does not depend on the shapes of the symbols. In our examples a filled up position is announced by the clenching of the right hand. An empty position is represented by the clenching of the left hand. The kinesthetic representation for both pictures is the clenching of the right hand once and the left hand once which is equal to a value of one.

GREEN LESSONS, LESSON 1, Figure 3

In Figure 3, we have a ***visual*** display of two pictures with two positions each. Both pictures have the same audio representations. The figures have different symbols in filled positions. In the first picture the second position is filled with two stars, and in second picture, a red ball. The shape and the number of symbols in the second position do not change the mathematical meaning.

The ***audio*** representation for both pictures consists of a **double knock and knock**, where a double knock represents an empty position and a knock represents a filled up position.

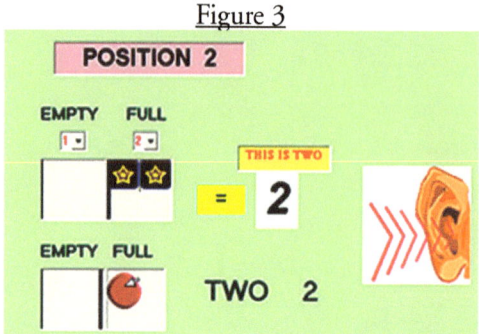

Figure 3

The ***kinesthetic*** representation of both figures does not depend on the shape or the number of the symbols in filled positions. In both pictures the filled position is represented by the clenching of the right hand. The empty position is represented by the clenching of the left hand. The kinesthetic representation for both pictures is the clenching of the left hand once and the right hand once, which is equal to a value of two.

GREEN LESSONS, LESSON 1, Figure 4

In Figure 4, we have a ***visual*** display of two pictures with two positions each. Both pictures have the same audio representations. In both pictures the two positions are filled with symbols. The first picture has stars in the filled positions and the second picture has red balls. In the first picture we have two positions filled with three stars. The shape and the number of the symbols in the picture do not change the mathematical meaning and correspond to the same audio signal. The ***audio*** representation for both pictures consists of **knock and knock**, where a knock is represents a filled position.

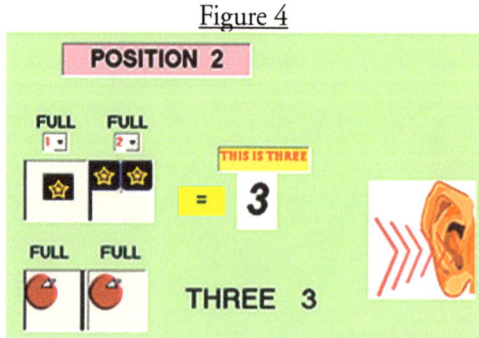

Figure 4

The ***kinesthetic*** representation of both figures does not depend on the shape and the number of the symbols in the filled positions. In both pictures the filled up position is represented by the clenching of the right hand twice, which is equal to a value of three.

GREEN LESSONS, LESSON 1, Figure 5

In Figure 5, we have a ***visual*** display of two pictures with three positions each. Both pictures have the same audio representations. The figures have different symbols in filled positions. There are four stars in the third position of the first picture and a red ball in the third position of the second picture. The shape and the number of the symbols in the third position of both pictures do not change the mathematical value. In both pictures the first two positions are empty and the third position is filled with a symbol.

The ***audio*** representation for both pictures consists of a **double knock, double knock and knock**, where double knock represents an empty position and knock represents a filled up position.

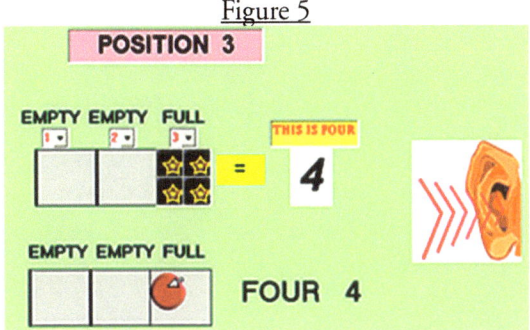

Figure 5

The ***kinesthetic*** representation of both figures does not depend on the shape and the number of the symbols in filled position. In both pictures the filled position three is represented by the clenching of the right hand. An empty position is represented by the clenching of the left hand. The **kinesthetic** representation for both pictures is the clenching of the left hand twice and the right hand once, which is equal to a value of four.

GREEN LESSONS, LESSON 1, Figure 6

In Figure 6, we have a ***visual*** display of two pictures with three positions each. Both pictures have the same audio representations. Positions one and three are filled with symbols. The first and third positions in the first picture are filled with stars and in the second picture, with red balls. In the first picture, the number of filled stars is equal to five. The shape and the number of symbols in the first and third positions of both pictures do not change the mathematical value.

The ***audio*** representation for both pictures consists of a **knock, double knock and knock**, where a knock represents a filled up position and a double knock represents an empty position.

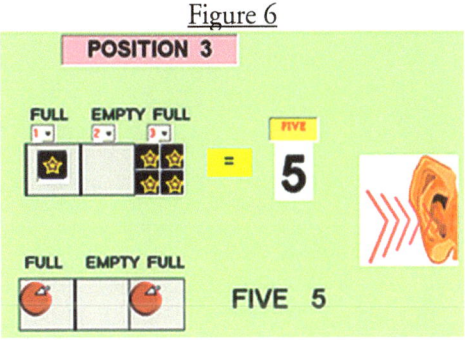

Figure 6

The ***kinesthetic*** representation of both figures does not depend on the shape or the number of symbols in the filled positions. In both pictures the first and third filled positions are represented by the clenching of the right hand. The empty position is represented by the clenching of the left hand. The kinesthetic representation for both pictures is the clenching of the right hand, left hand and right hand, which is equal to a value of four.

GREEN LESSONS, LESSON 1, Figure 7

In Figure 7, we have a *__visual__* display of two pictures with three positions each. Both pictures have the same audio representations. The second and third positions in the first pictures are filled with stars and the second and third positions in the second picture are filled with red balls. The shape and the number of symbols in second and third positions of both pictures do not change the mathematical meaning and have the same audio signals. In both pictures the first position is empty and the second and third positions are filled with a symbol.

The *__audio__* representation for both pictures consists of a **double knock, knocks and knock,** where a double knock represents an empty position and a knock represents a filled up position.

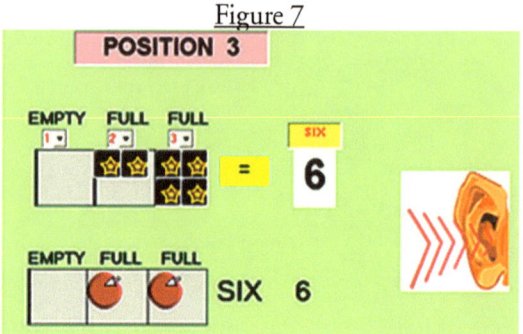

Figure 7

The *__kinesthetic__* representation of both figures does not depend on the shape or the number of the symbols. In both pictures, the second and third filled positions are represented by the clenching of the right hand twice. The empty position is represented by the clenching of the left hand. The kinesthetic representation for both pictures is the clenching of the left hand once and the right hand twice, which is equal to a value of six.

GREEN LESSONS, LESSON 1, Figure 8

In Figure 8, we have a *__visual__* display of two pictures with three positions each. Both pictures have the same audio representations. In both pictures all three positions are filled with symbols. The first picture is filled with seven stars and the second picture is filled with red balls. When we count the amount of the stars in the first picture, the number equals the mathematical value of the image. The shape and the number of the symbols in both pictures do not change the mathematical value. The *__audio__* representation for both pictures consists of **knock, knock and knocks**, where a knock represents a filled up position.

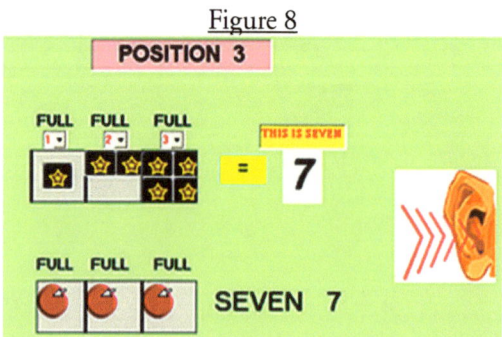

Figure 8

The *__kinesthetic__* representation of both figures does not depend on the shape or the number of the symbols in the filled positions. In both pictures the filled positions are represented by the clenching of the right hand three times, which is equal to a value of seven.

GREEN LESSONS, LESSON 1, Figure 9

In Figure 9, we have a ***visual*** display of two pictures with four positions each. The pictures have two different audio representations. The figures correspond to the visual representation of different numbers which are the combination of filled up and empty positions.

The ***audio*** representation of filled up positions is a knock. A double knock represents an empty position. In the first picture, we have four empty spaces and the audio illustration is **double knock, double knock, double knock and double knock**. In the second picture, only the fourth position is filled with a symbol and the positions one, two and three are empty. The audio representation for the second picture consists of a **double knock, double knock, double knock and knock**.

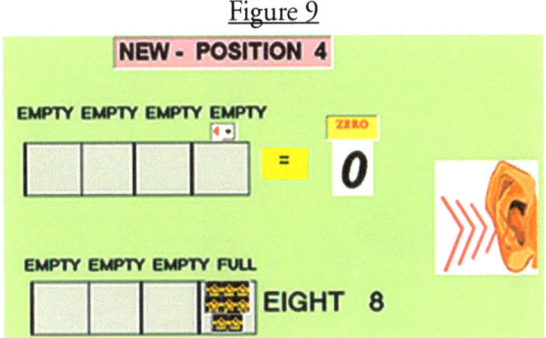

Figure 9

The ***kinesthetic*** representation of a filled up position is represented by the clenching of the right hand. An empty position is represented by the clenching of the left hand. The kinesthetic representation for the first picture is the clenching of the left hand four times, which is equal to a value of zero. The kinesthetic representation of the second picture is the clenching of the left hand three times, then the right hand once, which signifies a mathematical value equal to eight.

GREEN LESSONS, LESSON 1, Figure 10

In Figure 10, we have a ***visual*** display of two pictures with four positions each. The fourth position of the first picture is filled with eight balls and the fourth position of the second picture is filled with a red ball. The shape and the number of the symbols in fourth position do not change the mathematical meaning. In both pictures the first three positions are empty and the fourth position is filled with a symbol.

The ***audio*** representation for both pictures consists of a **double knock, double knock, double knock, and knock**, where a double knock represents an empty position and a knock represents a filled position.

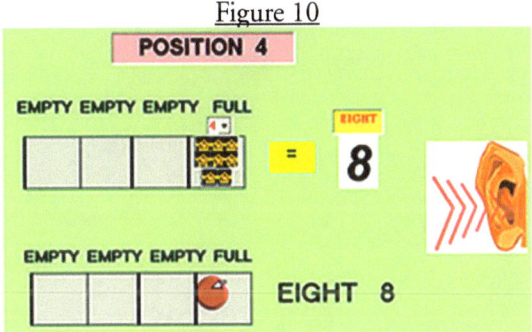

Figure 10

The ***kinesthetic*** representation of both figures does not depend on the shape or the number of the symbols in the filled position. In both pictures the filled position is represented by the clenching of the right hand. An empty position is represented by the clenching of the left hand. The kinesthetic representation for both pictures is the clenching of the left hand three times and the right hand once, which is equal to a value of eight.

GREEN LESSONS, LESSON 1, Figure 11

In Figure 11, we have a *__visual__* display of two pictures with four positions each. Both pictures have the same audio representations. In both pictures, positions one and four are filled with symbols. The first picture has one star in the first and eight stars in the fourth positions. The second picture has red balls in both first and fourth positions. The shape and the number of symbols in the first and forth positions of both pictures do not change the mathematical meaning. The *__audio__* representation for both pictures consists of a **knock, double knock, double knock and knock**, where a knock represents a filled up position and a double knock represents an empty position

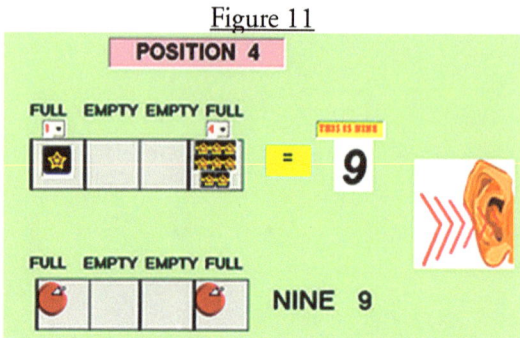

The *__kinesthetic__* representation of both figures does not depend on the shape or the number of the symbols in filled positions. In both pictures the filled first and fourth positions are represented by the clenching of the right hand. An empty position is represented by the clenching of the left hand. The kinesthetic representation for both pictures is the clenching of the right hand, then left hand twice and the right hand once, which is equal to a value of nine.

GREEN LESSONS, LESSON 1, Figure 12

In Figure 12, we have a *__visual__* display of two pictures with four positions each. Both pictures have the same audio representations. The second and fourth positions in the first picture are filled with two and eight stars, which is equal to a mathematical value of ten. The second and fourth positions of the second picture are filled with red balls. The shape and the number of the symbols in the second and forth positions of both pictures do not change the mathematical meaning. The *__audio__* representation for both pictures consists of a **double knock, knock, double knock and knock**, where a knock represents a filled up position and a double knock represents an empty position.

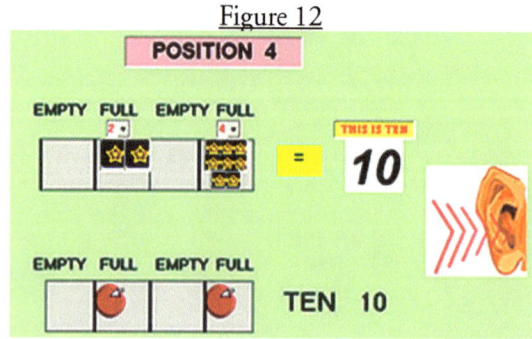

The *__kinesthetic__* representation of both figures does not depend on the shape or the number of the symbols in the filled positions. In both pictures the second and fourth filled positions are represented by the clenching of the right hand. An empty position is represented by the clenching of the left hand. The kinesthetic representation for both pictures is the clenching of the left hand, right, left and right, which is equal to a value of ten.

GREEN LESSONS, LESSON 2, Figure 1

In Figure 1, we have a *__visual__* display of two pictures with four positions each. Both pictures have the same audio representations. Positions one, two and four are filled with symbols. The first, second, and fourth positions in the first picture are filled with one, two, and eight stars. The number of stars corresponds to the mathematical value of the picture. The first, second, and fourth positions of the second picture are filled with red balls. The shape and the number of the symbols in the first, second and fourth positions of both pictures do not change the mathematical value.

The *__audio__* representation for both pictures consists of a **knock, knock, double knock and knock**, where a knock represents a filled up position and a double knock represents an empty position.

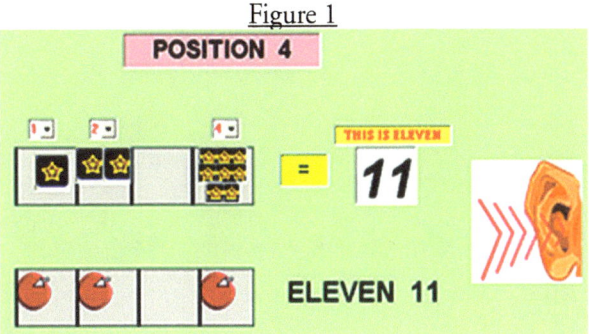

Figure 1

The *__kinesthetic__* representation of both figures does not depend on the shape or the number of the symbols in filled positions. In both pictures the first, second, and fourth filled positions are represented by the clenching of the right hand. An empty position is represented by the clenching of the left hand. The kinesthetic representation for both pictures is the clenching of the right hand twice, left once and again the right hand once, which is equal to a value of eleven.

GREEN LESSONS, LESSON 2, Figure 2

In Figure 2, we have a *__visual__* display of two pictures with four positions each. Both pictures have the same audio representations. In the first picture, in the filled positions we see twelve stars, and in the second picture we see two red balls. In both pictures the first two positions are empty and positions three and four are filled with symbols.

The *__audio__* representation for both pictures consists of a **double knock, double knock, knock and knock**, where a double knock represents an empty position and a knock represents a filled up position.

Figure 2

[Figure 2: POSITION 4 — shows visual with stars in positions 3 and 4, "= 12", "THIS IS TWELVE", and below red balls in positions 3 and 4 with "TWELVE 12"]

    The **_kinesthetic_** representation of both figures does not depend on the shape or the number of the symbols in the filled positions. In both pictures the filled up position is represented by the clenching of the right hand. An empty position is represented by the clenching of the left hand. The kinesthetic representation for both pictures is the clenching of the left hand twice and the right hand twice, which is equal to a value of twelve.

GREEN LESSONS, LESSON 2, Figure 3

    In Figure 3, we have a **_visual_** display of two pictures with four positions each. Both pictures have the same audio representations. In both pictures the first, third and fourth positions are filled with symbols. We have one star in the first position, four stars in the third position and eight stars in the fourth position. In the second picture in the first, third and forth positions are filled with a red ball. In the first picture the amount of stars is equal to thirteen. The shape and the number of the symbols in the first, third and forth positions of in pictures does not change the mathematical value. The **_audio_** representation for both pictures consists of a **knock, double knock, knock and knock,** where a knock represents a filled up position and a double knock represents an empty position.

Figure 3

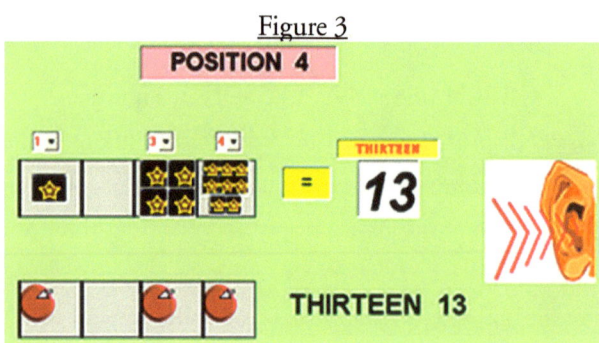

    The **_kinesthetic_** representation of both figures does not depend on the shape or the number of the symbols in filled positions. In both pictures the first, third, and fourth filled positions are represented by the clenching of the right hand. An empty position is represented by the clenching of the left hand. The kinesthetic representation for both pictures is the clenching of the right hand, left and the right hand twice, which is equal to a value of thirteen.

GREEN LESSONS, LESSON 2, Figure 4

In Figure 4, we have a *__visual__* display of two pictures with four positions each. Both pictures have the same audio representations. In the first picture, in filled up positions we see fourteen stars and in the second picture we see three red balls. The shape and the number of the symbols in second, third and fourth positions do not change the mathematical value.

The *__audio__* representation for both pictures consists of a **double knock, knock, knock and knock**, where a double knock represents an empty position and a knock represents a filled up position.

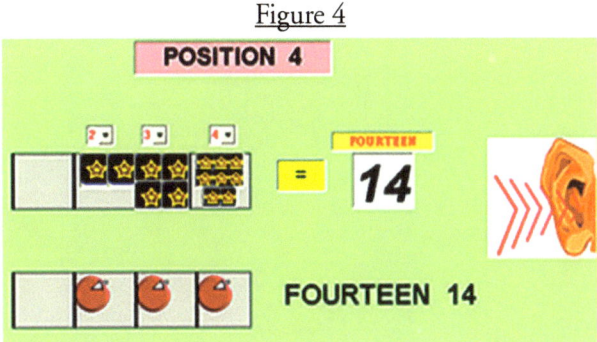

Figure 4

The *__kinesthetic__* representation of both figures does not depend on the shape or the number of symbols in filled positions. In both pictures the filled position is represented by the clenching of the right hand. An empty position is represented by the clenching of the left hand. The kinesthetic representation for both pictures is the clenching of the left hand once then the right hand three times, which is equal to a value of fourteen.

GREEN LESSONS, LESSON 2, Figure 5

In Figure 5, we have a *__visual__* display of two pictures with four positions each. Both pictures have the same audio representations. In both pictures all four positions are filled with symbols, but the figures have different symbols in the filled positions. In the first picture, we see fifteen stars and in the second picture we see four red balls. The shape and the number of the symbols in all positions do not change the mathematical value.

The *__audio__* representation for both pictures consists of a **knock, knock, knock and knock**, where a knock represents a filled up position.

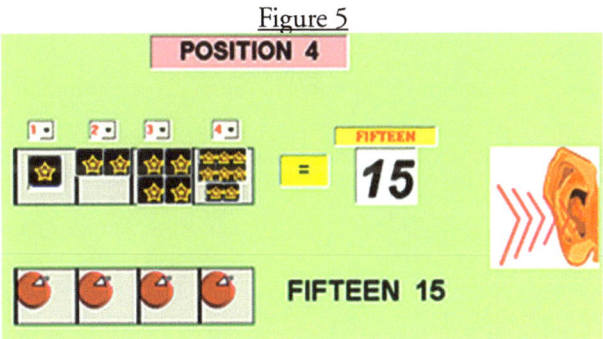

Figure 5

The *__kinesthetic__* representation of both figures does not depend on the shape or the number of symbols in the filled positions. In both pictures the filled position is represented by the clenching of the right hand four times, which is equal to a value of fifteen.

GREEN LESSONS, LESSON 3, Figure 1

In Figure 1, we have a *__visual__* display of two pictures with four positions each. The pictures have different audio representations.

The *__audio__* representation of a filled up position is a knock, and a double knock represents an empty position. In the first picture, we have five empty spaces and the audio representation is **double knock, double knock, double knock, double knock and double knock**. In the second picture, the fifth position is filled with a symbol and positions one, two, three, and four are empty. The audio representation for the second picture consists of a **double knock, double knock, double knock, double knock and knock**.

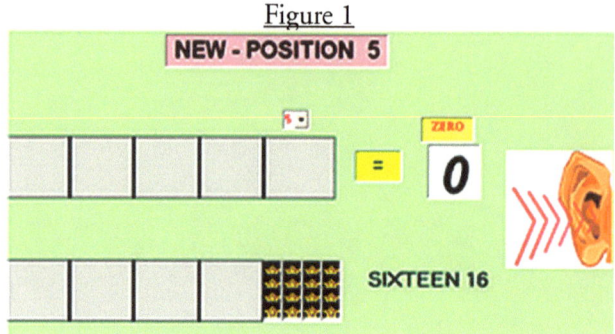

Figure 1

The *__kinesthetic__* representation of a filled up position is represented by the clenching of the right hand. An empty position is represented by the clenching of the left hand. The kinesthetic representation for the first picture is the clenching of the left hand five times, which is equal to zero. The kinesthetic representation of the second picture is the clenching of left hand four times, then the right hand once, which signifies a mathematical value equal to sixteen.

GREEN LESSONS, LESSON 3, Figure 3

In Figure 3, we have a *__visual__* display of two pictures with four positions each. Both pictures have the same audio representations. In both pictures position one and five are filled up with symbols. The figures have different symbols in filled positions. In the first picture, the first and fifth positions are filled with symbols. We have one star in the first position and sixteen stars in the forth position. In the second picture, there is a red ball in the first and fifth positions. The shape and the number of symbols in the first and fifth positions of both pictures do not change the mathematical value. The *__audio__* representation for both pictures consists of a **knock, double knock, double knock, double knock and knock**, where a knock represents a filled up position and a double knock represents an empty position.

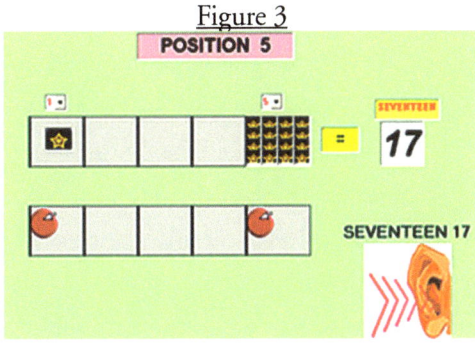

Figure 3

The ***kinesthetic*** representation of both figures does not depend on the shape and the number of symbols in the filled positions. In both pictures the first and fifth filled positions are represented by the clenching of the right hand. An empty position is represented by the clenching of the left hand. The kinesthetic representation for both pictures is the clenching of the right hand, then left hand three times and the right hand once, which is equal to a value of seventeen.

GREEN LESSONS, LESSON 3, Figure 4

In Figure 4, we have a ***visual*** display of two pictures with four positions each. Both pictures have the same audio representations. In both pictures position two and five are filled with symbols. The figures have different symbols in filled positions. In the first picture, the second and fifth positions are filled with symbols. We have two stars in the second position and sixteen stars in the fifth position. In the second picture, there is a red ball in the second and fifth positions. The shape and the number of the symbols in the second and fifth positions of both pictures do not change the mathematical value. The ***audio*** representation for both pictures consists of a **double knock, knock, double knock, double knock and knock**, where a knock represents a filled up position and a double knock represents an empty position.

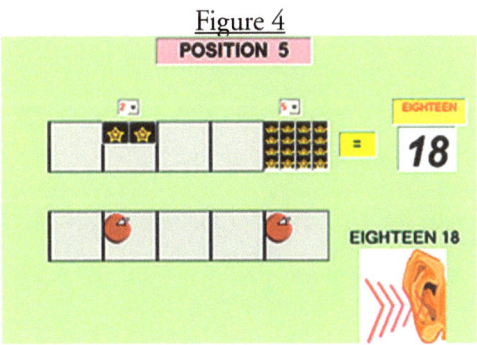

Figure 4

The ***kinesthetic*** representation of both figures does not depend on the shape or the number of symbols in the filled positions. In both pictures the second and fifth filled positions are represented by the clenching of the right hand. An empty position is represented by the clenching of the left hand. The kinesthetic representation for both pictures is the clenching of the left hand, right, left twice and right again, which is equal to a value of eighteen.

GREEN LESSONS, LESSON 3, Figure 5

In Figure 5, we have a *__visual__* display of two pictures with four positions each. Both pictures have the same audio representations. The figures have different symbols in filled up positions. In the first picture, the first, second and fifth positions are filled with symbols. We have one star in the first position, two stars in the second position and sixteen stars in the fifth position. In the second picture, the first, second and fifth positions are filled with red balls. The shape and the number of symbols in the first, second and fifth positions of both pictures do not change the mathematical value. The *__audio__* representation for both pictures consists of a **knock, knock, double knock, double knock and knock**, where a knock represents a filled up position and a double knock represents an empty position.

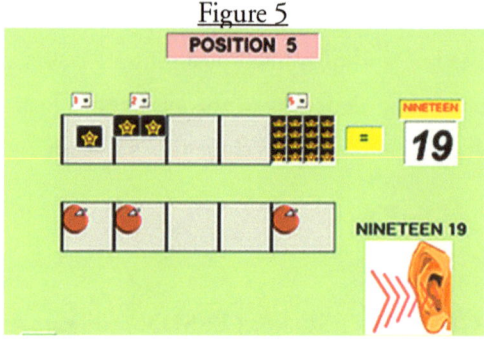

Figure 5

The *__kinesthetic__* representation of both figures does not depend on the shape and the number of symbols in the filled positions. The first, second and fifth filled positions are filled with symbols represented by the clenching of the right hand. An empty position is represented by the clenching of the left hand. The kinesthetic representation for both pictures is the clenching of the right hand twice, left twice and the right hand again, which is equal to a value of nineteen.

GREEN LESSONS, LESSON 3, Figure 6

In Figure 6, we have a *__visual__* display of two pictures with four positions each. Both pictures have the same audio representations. The figures have different symbols in filled positions. In the first picture, the third and fifth positions are filled with symbols. We have four stars in the third position and sixteen stars in the fifth position. In the second picture, there are red balls in third and fifth positions. The shape and the number of symbols in the third and fifth positions of both pictures do not change the mathematical value. The *__audio__* representation for both pictures consists of a **double knock, double knock, knock, double knock and knock**, where a knock represents a filled up position and a double knock represents an empty position.

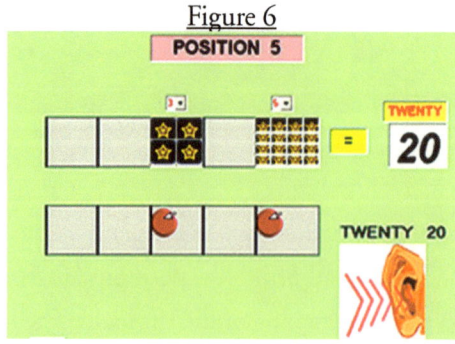

Figure 6

The *__kinesthetic__* representation of both figures does not depend on the shape or the number of the symbols in the filled positions. In both pictures the third and fifth filled positions are represented by the clenching of the right hand. An empty position is represented by the clenching of the left hand. The kinesthetic representation for both pictures is the clenching of the left twice, right, left and right again, which is equal to a value of twenty.

GREEN LESSONS, LESSON 4, Figure 1

In Figure 1, the **_visual_** display of both pictures has five positions each. Both pictures have the same audio representation. The figures have different symbols in filled positions. In the first picture the first, third and fifth positions are filled with symbols. We have one star in the first position, four stars in the in third position and sixteen stars in the fifth position. In the second picture, there are red balls in the first, third, and fifth positions. The shape and the number of symbols in the first, third and fifth positions in both pictures do not change the mathematical value. The **_audio_** representation for both pictures consists of a **knock, double knock, knock, double knock and knock** where a knock represents a filled position and a double knock represents an empty position

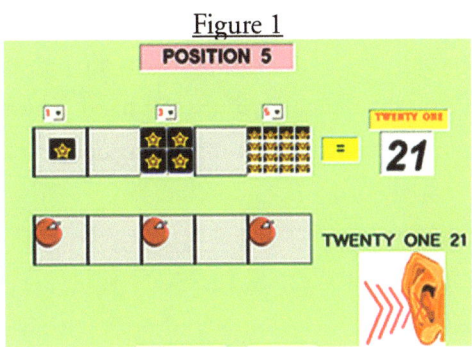

Figure 1

The **_kinesthetic_** representation of both figures does not depend on the shape or the number of symbols in the filled positions. The first, third, and fifth filled positions in the picture are represented by the clenching of the right hand. An empty position is represented by the clenching of the left hand. The kinesthetic representation for both pictures is the clenching of the right hand, left, right, left and right again, which is equal to a value of twenty one.

GREEN LESSONS, LESSON 4, Figure 2

In Figure 2, we have a **_visual_** display of two pictures with four positions each. Both pictures have the same audio representations. The figures have different symbols in filled positions. In the first picture the second, third and fifth positions are filled with symbols. We have two stars in the second position, four stars in the in third position and sixteen stars in the fifth position. In the second picture, there are red balls in the second, third, and fifth positions. The shape and the number of symbols in the second, third and fifth positions in both pictures do not change the mathematical value. The **_audio_** representation for both pictures consists of a **double knock, knock, knock, double knock and knock,** where a knock represents a filled up position and a double knock represents an empty position.

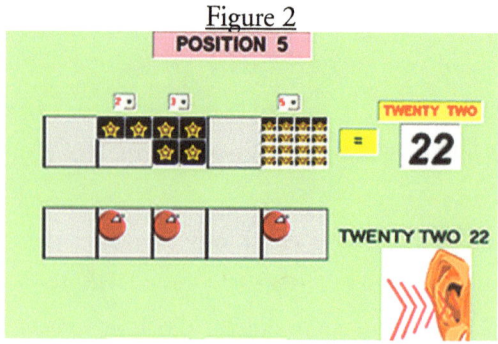

Figure 2

The **_kinesthetic_** representation of both figures does not depend on the shape or the number of filled positions. In both pictures the second, third, and fifth filled positions are represented by the clenching of the right hand. An empty position is represented by the clenching of the left hand. The kinesthetic representation for both pictures is the clenching of the left hand, right twice, left and right again, which is equal to a value of twenty two.

GREEN LESSONS, LESSON 4, Figure 3

In Figure 3, we have a **_visual_** display of two pictures with four positions each. Both pictures have the same audio representations. The figures have different symbols in filled positions. The first, second, third, and fifth positions in the first picture are filled with stars, and the number of the stars adds up to twenty three. The first, second, third, and fifth positions in the second picture are filled with red balls. The shape and the number of the symbols in the first, second, third and fifth positions in both pictures do not change the mathematical value. The **_audio_** representation for both pictures consists of a **knock, knock, knock, double knock and knock,** where a knock represents a filled position and a double knock represents an empty position.

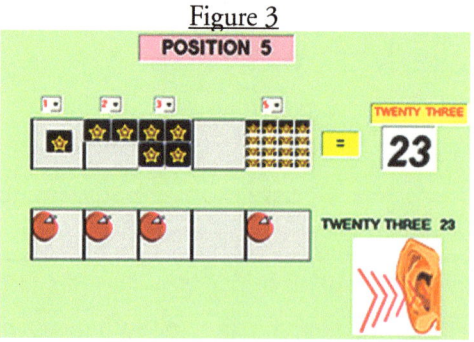

Figure 3

The **_kinesthetic_** representation of both figures does not depend on the shape or the number of symbols in the filled positions. In both pictures, the first, second, third, and fifth filled positions are represented by the clenching of the right hand. An empty position is represented by the clenching of the left hand. The kinesthetic representation for both pictures is the clenching of the right hand three times, left once and right once more, which is equal to a value of twenty three.

GREEN LESSONS, LESSON 4, Figure 4

In Figure 4, we have a ***visual*** display of two pictures with four positions each. Both pictures have the same audio representations. The figures have different symbols in filled positions. The fourth and fifth positions in the first picture are filled with twenty four stars, and the fourth and fifth positions in the second picture are filled with red balls. The shape and the number of the symbols in the filled positions do not change the mathematical value. In both pictures the first three positions are empty, and positions four and five are filled with a symbol.

The ***audio*** representation for both pictures consists of a **double knock, double knock, double knock, knock and knock**, where a double knock represents an empty position and a knock represents a filled up position.

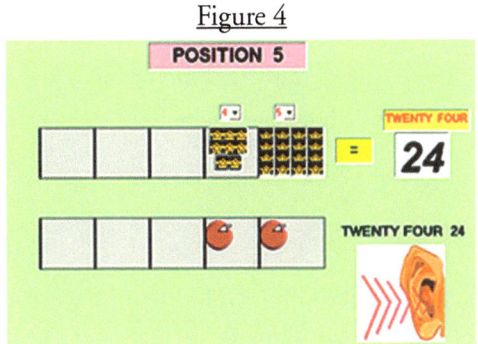

Figure 4

The ***kinesthetic*** representation of both figures does not depend on the shape or the number of the symbols in the filled positions. In both pictures the filled position is represented by the clenching of the right hand. An empty position is represented by the clenching of the left hand. The kinesthetic representation for both pictures is the clenching of the left hand three times and the right hand twice, which is equal to a value of twenty four.

GREEN LESSONS, LESSON 4, Figure 5

In Figure 5, we a have ***visual*** display of two pictures with four positions each. Both pictures have the same audio representations. The figures have different symbols in filled positions. The first, fourth, and fifth positions in the first picture are filled with twenty five stars, and the same positions in the second picture are filled with red balls. The shape and the number of symbols in the first, fourth and fifth positions in both pictures do not change the mathematical value.

The ***audio*** representation for both pictures consists of a **knock, double knock, double knock, knock and knock**, where a knock represents a filled up position and a double knock represents an empty position.

Figure 5

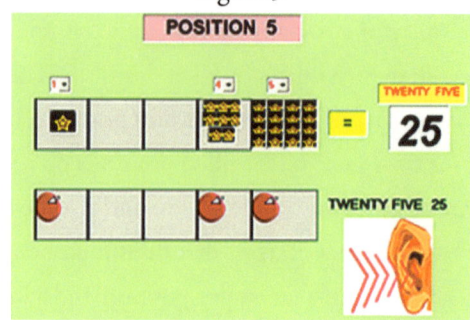

The ***kinesthetic*** representation of both figures does not depend on the shape or the number of symbols in the filled positions. In both pictures, the first, fourth, and fifth filled positions are represented by the clenching of the right hand. An empty position is represented by the clenching of the left hand. The kinesthetic representation for both pictures is the clenching of the right hand, left twice, and the right hand twice, which is equal to a value of twenty five.

GREEN LESSONS, LESSON 4, Figure 1

In Figure 1, we have a ***visual*** display of two pictures with four positions each. Both pictures have the same audio representations. The figures have different symbols in filled positions. The second, fourth, and fifth positions in the first picture are filled with twenty six stars, and the same positions in the second picture are filled with red balls. The shape and the number of symbols in the second, fourth and fifth positions in both pictures do not change the mathematical value. The ***audio*** representation for both pictures consists of a **double knock, knock, double knock, knock and knock,** where a knock represents a filled position and a double knock represents an empty position.

Figure 1

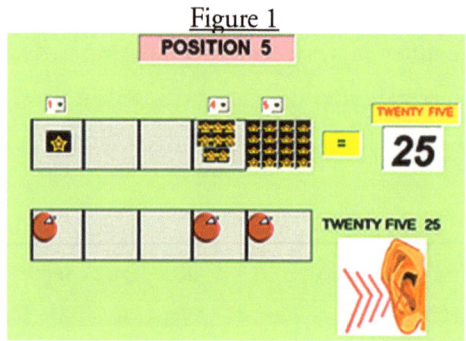

The ***kinesthetic*** representation of both figures does not depend on the shape or the number of symbols in the filled positions. In both pictures, the second, fourth, and fifth filled positions are represented by the clenching of the right hand. An empty position is represented by the clenching of the left hand. The kinesthetic representation for both pictures is the clenching of the left hand, right, left and right hand twice, which is equal to a value of twenty six.

GREEN LESSONS, LESSON 4, Figure 2

In Figure 3, we have a ***visual*** display of two pictures with four positions each. Both pictures have the same audio representations. The figures have different symbols in filled positions. The first, second, fourth and fifth positions in the first picture are filled with twenty seven stars, and the same positions in the second picture are filled with red balls. The shape and the number of symbols in the first, second, fourth and fifth positions in both pictures do not change the mathematical value.

The ***audio*** representation for both pictures consists of a **knock, knock, double knock, knock, knock,** where a knock represents a filled up position and a double knock represents an empty position.

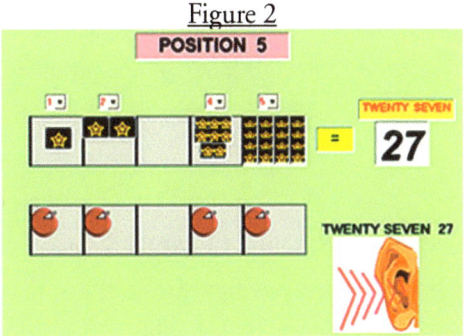

Figure 2

The ***kinesthetic*** representation of both figures does not depend on the shape or the number of symbols in the filled positions. In both pictures, the first, second, fourth, and fifth filled positions are represented by the clenching of the right hand. An empty position is represented by the clenching of the left hand. The kinesthetic representation for both pictures is the clenching of the right hand twice, left once and right twice again, which is equal to a value of twenty seven.

GREEN LESSONS, LESSON 5, Figure 3

In Figure 3, we have a ***visual*** display of two pictures with four positions each. Both pictures have the same audio representations. The figures have different symbols in filled positions. The third, fourth, and fifth positions in the first picture are filled with twenty eight stars, and the same positions in the second picture are filled with red balls. The shape and the number of symbols in the filled positions do not change the mathematical value.

The ***audio*** representation for both pictures consists of a **double knock, double knock, knock, knock and knock**, where a double knock represents an empty position and a knock represents a filled up position.

Figure 3

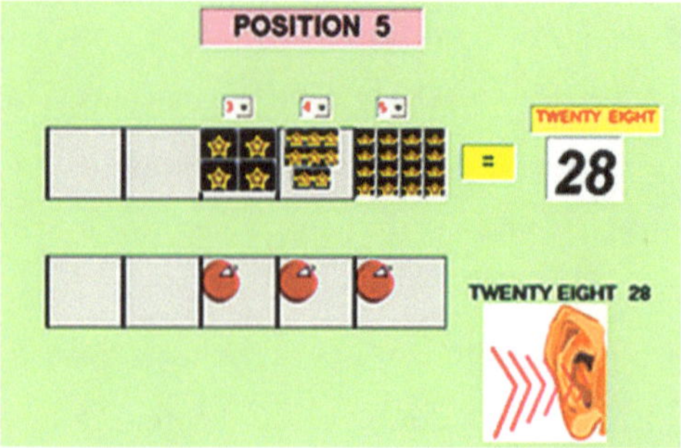

The ***kinesthetic*** representation of both figures does not depend on the shape or the number of symbols in the filled positions. In both pictures, the filled positions are represented by the clenching of the right hand. An empty position is represented by the clenching of the left hand. The kinesthetic representation for both pictures is the clenching of the left hand two times and the right hand three times, which is equal to a value of twenty eight.

GREEN LESSONS, LESSON 5, Figure 4

In Figure 3, we have a ***visual*** display of two pictures with four positions each. Both pictures have the same audio representations. The figures have different symbols in the filled positions. The first, third, fourth, and fifth positions in the first picture are filled with twenty nine stars, and the same positions in the second picture are filled with red balls. The shape and the number of symbols in the first, third, fourth and fifth positions of both pictures do not change the mathematical value.

The ***audio*** representation for both pictures consists of a **knock, double knock, knock, knock and knock**, where a knock represents a filled up position and a double knock represents an empty position.

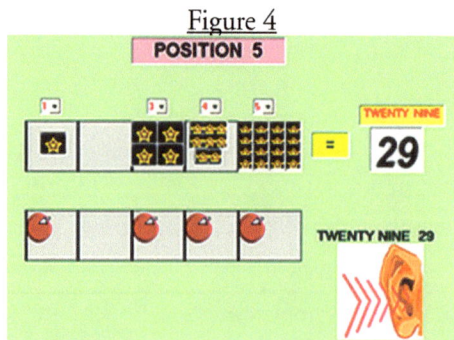

Figure 4

The ***kinesthetic*** representation of both figures does not depend on the shape or the number of symbols in the filled positions. In both pictures, the filled up positions are represented by the clenching of the right hand. An empty position is represented by the clenching of the left hand. The kinesthetic representation for both pictures is the clenching of the right hand, left and the right hand three times, which is equal to a value of twenty nine.

GREEN LESSONS, LESSON 5, Figure 5

In Figure 5, we have a *__visual__* display of two pictures with four positions each. Both pictures have the same audio representations. The figures have different symbols in the filled positions. The second, third, fourth and fifth positions in the first picture are filled with thirty stars, and the same positions in the second picture are filled with red balls. The shape or the number of symbols in the filled positions does not change the mathematical value.

The *__audio__* representation for both pictures consists of a **double knock, knock, knock, knock and knock**, where a double knock represents an empty position and a knock represents a filled up position.

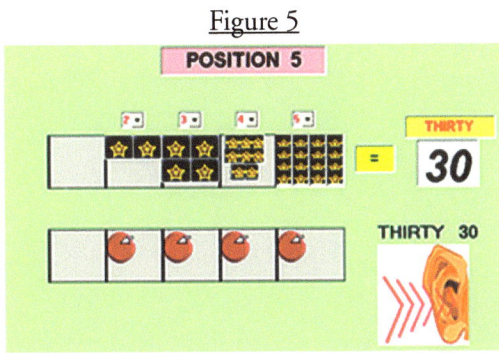

Figure 5

The *__kinesthetic__* representation of both figures does not depend on the shape or the number of symbols in the filled positions. In both pictures, the filled positions are represented by the clenching of the right hand. An empty position is represented by the clenching of the left hand. The kinesthetic representation for both pictures is the clenching of the left hand once and the right hand four times, which is equal to a value of thirty.

GREEN LESSONS, LESSON 5, Figure 6

In Figure 6, we have a *__visual__* display of two pictures with four positions each. Both pictures have the same audio representations. In both pictures all five positions are filled with symbols. The first picture is filled with stars and the second is filled with red balls. The shape and the number of symbols in all positions do not change the mathematical value.

The *__audio__* representation for both pictures consists of a **knock, knock, knock, knock and knock**, where a knock represents a filled position.

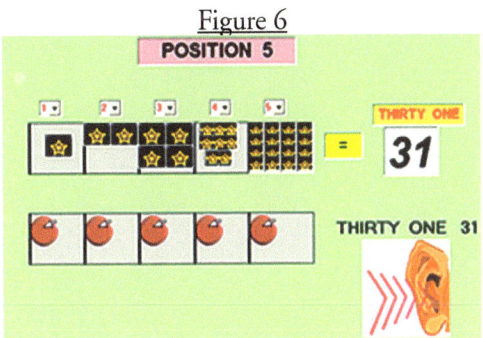

Figure 6

The *__kinesthetic__* representation of both figures does not depend on the shape or the number of symbols in the filled positions. In both pictures the filled positions are represented by the clenching of the right hand five times, which is equal to a value of thirty one.

MATHEMATICS

Count number of objects in

Each Picture

BLUE LESSONS, Figure 1

In Figure 1, we have a **<u>video</u>** display of two pictures with two positions each, where position one is filled up with symbols and the second position is empty. The **<u>audio</u>** representation of those figures is **knock and double knock**.

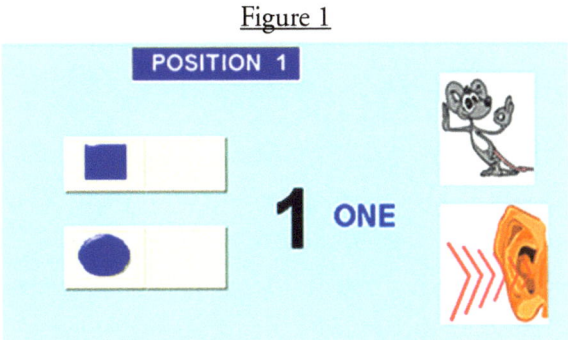

Figure 1

The knock represents the filled up position and double knock represents an empty position. In our example, the **<u>audio</u>** signals knock and double knock correspond to the both pictures. The first picture of boxes has a **<u>visual</u>** display of the square symbol in the first box and empty space in the second box. In the first position of the second picture includes a circle and the second position has an empty space. The different symbols in the first positions of the pictures do not change the mathematical representation of both configurations. The shape of the symbols also does not have any effect on the mathematical meaning. The symbols exist just to show that positions are already filled up. The mathematical value of the both first and second configurations is equal to one. Any shape of the symbols in the first position represents number one.

The **<u>kinesthetic</u>** representation of the knock is the clenching of the right hand and for double knock is the tightening the left hand into a fist. The filled up position is represented by the clenching of the right hand and an empty position represented by the clenching of the left hand. The **<u>kinesthetic</u>** representation for the first and second configurations of boxes is the clenching of the right and then the left hand.

BLUE LESSONS, Figure 2

Figure 2 is the **<u>visual</u>** display of two pictures with two positions each, where position one is empty and the second position is filled up with symbols. The **<u>audio</u>** representation of this figure is **double knock and knock**

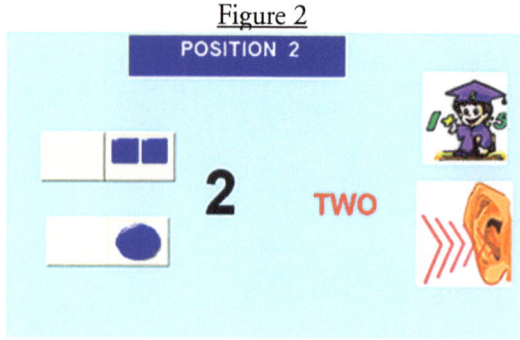

Figure 2

The double knock is the **audio** representation of the empty position and knock represents a filled up position. In our example double knock and knock correspond to both pictures. The first picture has an empty space in the first position and square symbol in the second. In the second picture, we see an empty space in the first positions and a circle in the second. The different **visual** shape of symbols in the second position does not change the mathematical meaning. The presence of the symbol is only to show that the position is already filled up. The mathematical value of the first configuration as well as the second is equal to two. Any shape of symbols in the second position represents number two. The **kinesthetic** representation of the double knock is the tightening of the left hand into a fist and for knock is the clenching of the right hand. An empty position is represented by the clenching of the left hand. The filled up position is represented by the clenching of the right hand. The **kinesthetic** representation for the first and second configurations of boxes is the clenching of the left hand and then the right.

BLUE LESSONS, Figure 3

In Figure 3, we have a **visual** presentation of two pictures with two positions each, where both positions are filled up with symbols. The **audio** representation of this figure is **knock and knock**.

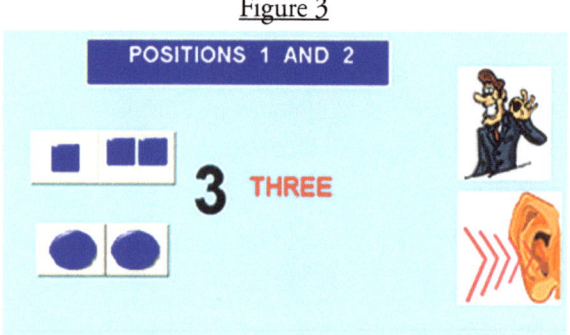

Figure 3

The two pictures correspond to the same mathematical value of number three. In our example, the **audio** signals knock and knock correspond to both pictures. The **visual** display of the first picture has a square symbol in both positions, where in first position is only one square and in the second position we have two squares. In the second picture we have circles in both positions. The different symbols in the first position do not change the mathematical representation of both configurations. The shape of the symbols does not affect the mathematical meaning. The symbols exist just to show that positions are already filled up. The one box in the first position and two boxes in the second position of the first picture are visually illustrating the mathematical quantity.

The **kinesthetic** representation of filled up positions is the clenching of the right hand. The **kinesthetic** representation for both pictures is the clenching of the right hand twice.

The two boxes in the second position of the first picture are **visually** illustrating the quantity of the mathematical representation.

BLUE LESSONS, Figure 4

In Figure 4, we have a **<u>visual</u>** representation of two pictures where each one has three positions. In both pictures positions one and two are empty. Only position three is filled up with a symbol. The ***audio*** representation of these figures is **double knock, double knock and knock**.

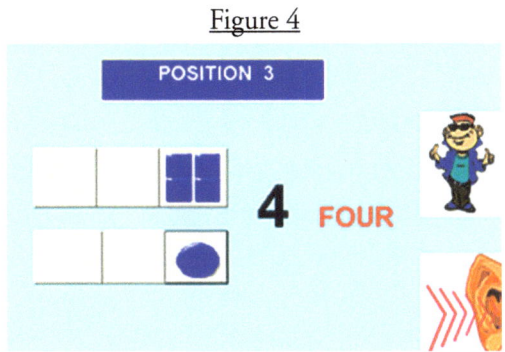

Figure 4

In the first and second positions of both pictures we have an empty space. In the third position we have rectangles or a circle. The different symbols in the third position of the pictures do not change the mathematical representation of both configurations. The shape of the symbols also does not affect the mathematical value. The symbols exist just to show that positions are already filled up. The mathematical value of the first and second configurations is equal to four.

The ***<u>kinesthetic</u>*** representation of the knock is the clenching of the right hand and for double knock is the tightening the left hand into a fist. The filled up position is represented by the clenching of the left hand two times and then by the clenching of the right hand.

BLUE LESSONS, Figure 5

In Figure 5 we have a **<u>visual</u>** display of two pictures, which have three positions each. The first and third positions are filled up with symbols. The second position is left empty. The **<u>audio</u>** representation of this figure is **knock, double knock, and knock**.

Figure 5

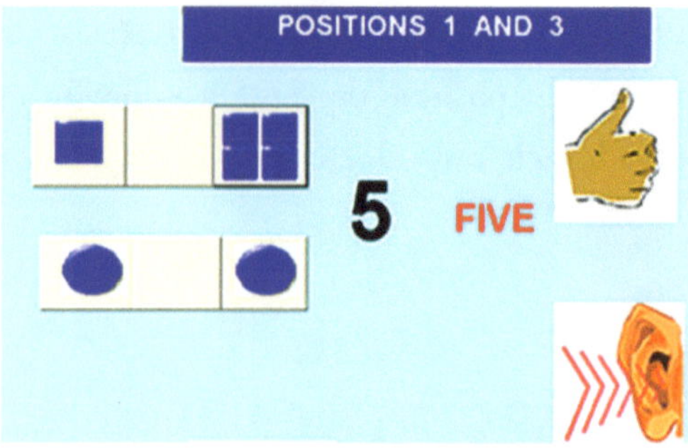

Pictures in boxes correspond to the mathematical value of number five.
The filled up position is represented by the **audio** signal of a knock, and an empty position is represented by a double knock. In our example knock, double knock, and knock correspond to both pictures. The first picture of boxes has a **visual** square symbol in the first and third place, but empty space in the second place. The different symbols in the first position of the pictures do not change the mathematical representation of both configurations. The shape of the symbols also does not affect the mathematical meaning. The symbols exist just to show that positions are already filled up. The **kinesthetic** representation of the knock is the clenching of the right hand and for double knock is the tightening of the left hand into a fist. The **kinesthetic** representation for the first and second configurations of boxes is the clenching of the right, left and right hand again.

BLUE LESSONS, Figure 6

In Figure 6, we have a **visual** display of two pictures with three positions each. Position one is empty, but position two and position three are filled up with symbols. The **audio** representation of those figures is **double knock, knock and knock**.

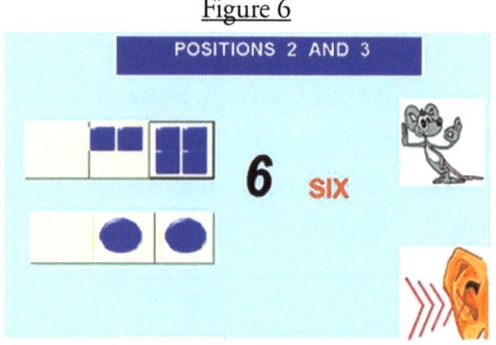

Figure 6

Pictures of boxes correspond to the mathematical value of number six.
The **audio** signal of a knock represents the **video** image of a filled up position and double knock represents an empty position. In our example double knock, knock and knock correspond to both pictures. The first picture of boxes has square symbols in the second and third place, but empty space in the first place. In the first position of the second picture we see an empty space and in the second and third positions we see a circle. The shape of the symbols does not affect the mathematical meaning. The symbols exist just to show that positions are already filled up. The mathematical value of the first configuration as well as the second is equal to six. The kinesthetic representation of the knock is the clenching of the right hand and for double knock is the tightening of the left hand into a fist. The **kinesthetic** representation for the first and second configurations of boxes is the clenching of the left hand once and the clenching the right hand twice.

BLUE LESSONS, Figure 7

In Figure 7 we have the **video** display of two pictures, which have three positions each. All positions are filled up with symbols. The **audio** representation of this figure is **knock, knock and knock**.

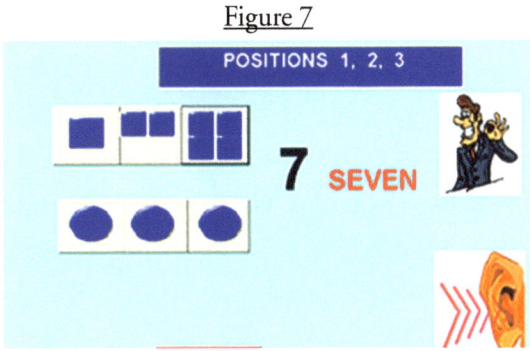

Figure 7

The **audio** signal of knock represents the filled up position and double knock represents an empty position. The **video** display of the first picture of boxes has square symbols in all places. In all positions of the second picture we see a circle. The different symbols in the first position of the pictures do not change the mathematical representation of both configurations. The shape of the symbols also does not affect the mathematical meaning. The symbols exist just to show that positions are already filled up. The mathematical value of the first configuration as well as the second is equal to seven. The **kinesthetic** representation of the knock is the clenching of the right hand and for double knock is the tightening of the left hand into a fist. The filled up position is represented by the clenching of the right hand and an empty position represented by the clenching of the left hand. The **kinesthetic** representation for the first and second configurations of boxes is the clenching of the right hand three times.

BLUE LESSONS, Figure 8

In Figure 8 we have a **visual** display of two pictures with four positions each. Positions one through three are empty and position four is filled up with symbols. The **audio** representation of those figures is **double knock, double knock, double knock and knock**.

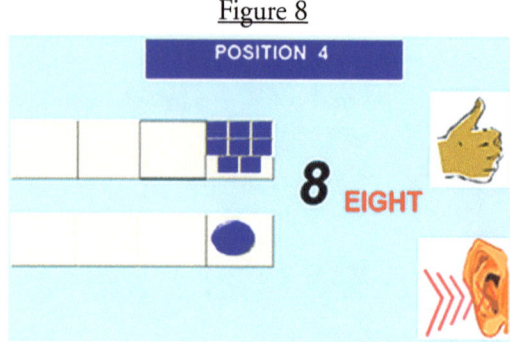

Figure 8

The **audio** signal of knock represents a filled up position and double knock represents an empty position. The **video** display of the first picture of boxes has a square symbol in the fourth place and empty spaces in the first place through third place. In the fourth position of the second picture we see a circle, but in the first, second, and third positions we have empty space. The shape of the symbols does not affect the mathematical meaning. The symbols exist just to show that positions are already filled up. The mathematical value of the first configuration as well as the second is equal to eight.

The kinesthetic representation of the knock is the clenching of the right hand and for double knock is the clenching of the left. The filled up position is represented by the clenching of the right hand and an empty position represented by the clenching of the left hand. The **kinesthetic** representation for the first and second configurations of boxes is the clenching of the left hand three times and then the right hand once.

BLUE LESSONS, Exercise, Figure 1

There is a combination of positions, filled up with symbols or empty spaces. In Figure 1 the audio representation of one of the pictures below is **knock and double knock**.

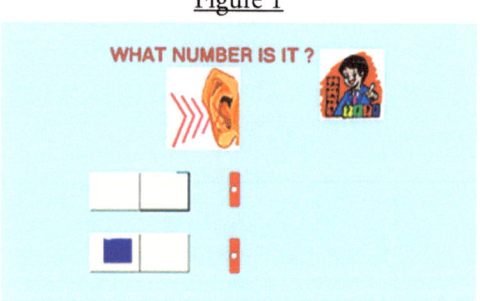

Figure 1

A knock represents a filled up position and a double knock represents an empty position. The clenching of the right hand represents a filled up position and the clenching of the left hand represents an empty position. The **kinesthetic** representation for the answer which corresponds to the second picture is the clenching of the right hand and left hand. The kinesthetic representation for the first picture is the clenching of the left hand twice.

BLUE LESSONS, EXERCISE, Figure 2

In Figure 2, we have three pictures with *__visual__* combinations of filled up symbols or empty spaces. The *__audio__* representation of one of the pictures below is **double knock and knock**

Figure 2

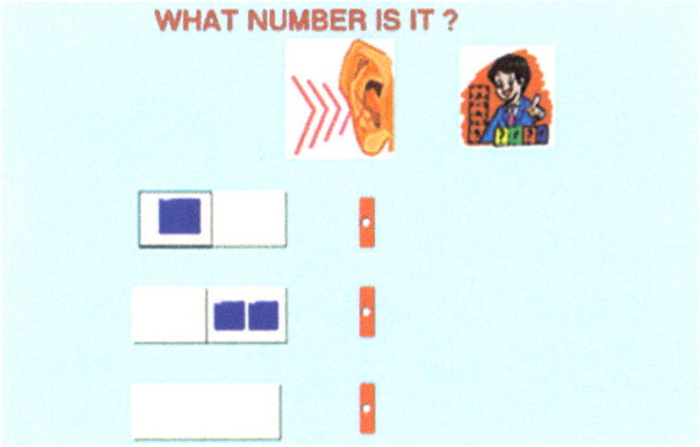

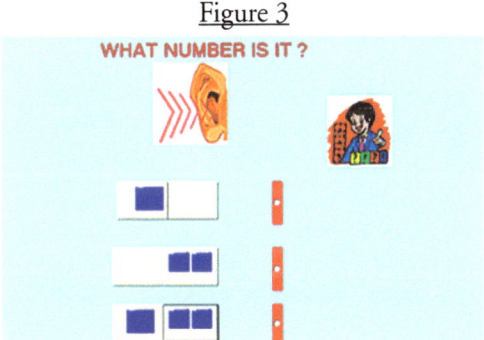

A knock represents a filled up position and a double knock represents an empty position. The clenching of the right hand represents a filled up position and the clenching of the left hand represents an empty position. The *__kinesthetic__* representation for the answer which corresponds to the second picture is the clenching of the left hand and right hand. The kinesthetic representation for the first picture is the clenching of the right hand and left hand. The kinesthetic representation for the third picture is the clenching of the left hand twice.

BLUE LESSONS, EXERCISE, Figure 3

In Figure 3, we have three different *__visual__* combinations of positions, filled up with symbols or empty positions. The *__audio__* representation of one of the pictures below is represented by **knock, knock.**

Figure 3

A knock represents a filled up position and a double knock represents an empty position. The clenching of the right hand represents a filled up position and the clenching of the left hand represents an empty position. The *__kinesthetic__* representation for the answer which corresponds to the third picture is the clenching of the right hand twice. The kinesthetic representation for the first picture is the clenching of the right hand and left hand. The kinesthetic representation for the second picture is the clenching of the left hand and right hand.

BLUE LESSONS, EXERCISE, Figure 4

In Figure 4, we have three *__visual__* combinations, filled up with symbols or empty positions. The *__audio__* representation of one of the pictures below is **double knock, double knock, and knock**.

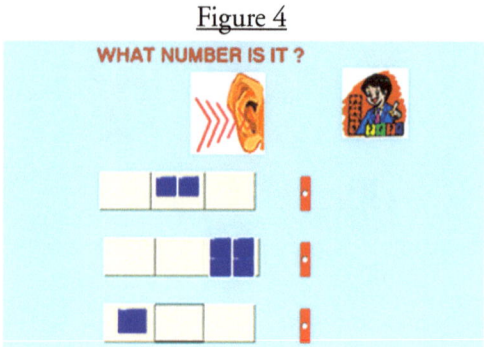

Figure 4

A knock represents a filled up position and a double knock represents an empty position. The clenching of the right hand represents a filled up position and the clenching of the left hand represents an empty position. The *__kinesthetic__* representation for the answer corresponding to the second picture is the clenching of the left hand twice and right hand. The kinesthetic representation for the first picture is the clenching of the left hand and right hand. The kinesthetic representation for the third picture is the clenching of the right hand and left hand twice.

BLUE LESSONS, EXERCISE, Figure 5

In Figure 5, we have three *__visual__* combinations, filled up with symbols or empty positions. The *__audio__* representation of one of the pictures below is **knock, double knock and knock**.

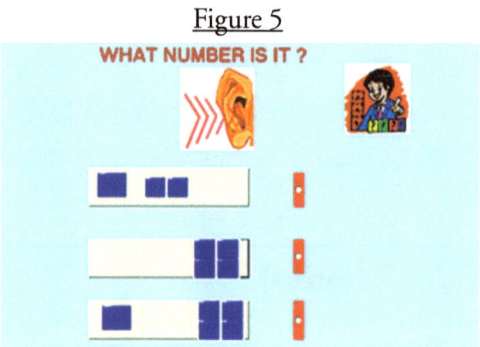

Figure 5

A knock represents a filled up position and a double knock represents an empty position. The clenching of the right hand represents a filled up position and the clenching of the left represents an empty position. The *__kinesthetic__* representation for the answer which corresponds to the third picture is the clenching of the right hand, left hand, and right hand. The kinesthetic representation for the first picture is the clenching of the right hand twice and left hand. The kinesthetic representation for the second picture is the clenching of the left hand twice and right hand.

BLUE LESSONS, EXERCISE, Figure 6

In Figure 6, we have three **_visual_** combinations, filled up with symbols or empty positions. The **_audio_** representation for one of the pictures below is **double knock, knock, and knock**.

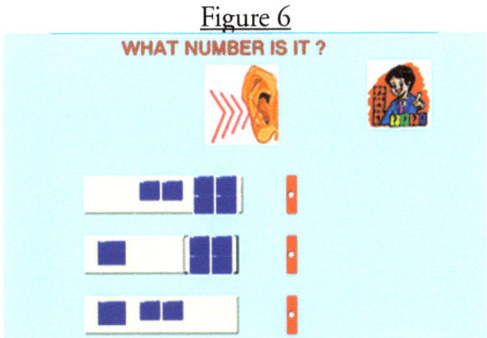

Figure 6

A knock represents a filled up position and a double knock represents an empty position. The clenching of the right hand represents a filled up position and the clenching of the left hand represents an empty position. The **_kinesthetic_** representation for the answer which corresponds to the first picture is the clenching of the left hand and right hand twice. The kinesthetic representation for the second picture is the clenching of the right hand, left hand, and right hand. The kinesthetic representation for the third picture is the clenching of the right hand twice and left hand.

BLUE LESSONS, EXERCISE, Figure 7

In Figure 7, we have three **_visual_** combinations that are filled up with symbols or empty positions. The **_audio_** representation of one of the pictures below is **knock, knock, and knock**.

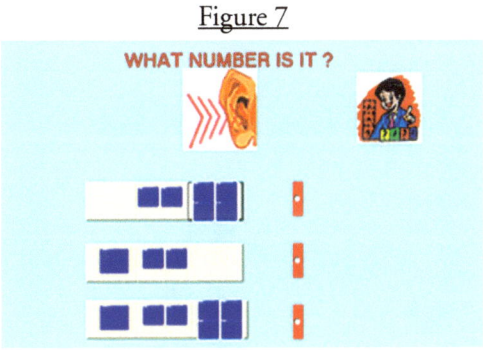

Figure 7

A knock represents a filled up position and a double knock represents an empty position. The clenching of the right hand represents a filled up position and the clenching of the left hand represents an empty position. The **_kinesthetic_** representation for the answer which corresponds to the third picture is the clenching of the right hand thrice. The kinesthetic representation for the first picture is the clenching of the left hand and right hand twice. The kinesthetic representation for the second picture is the clenching of the right hand twice and left hand.

BLUE LESSONS, EXERCISE, Figure 8

In Figure 8, we have three **_visual_** combinations that are filled up with symbols or empty positions. The **_audio_** representation of one of the pictures below is **double knock, double knock, double knock, and knock**.

Figure 8

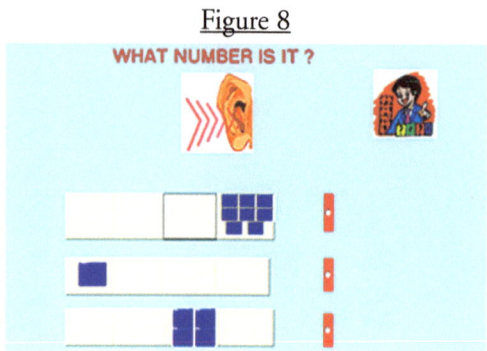

A knock represents a filled up position and a double knock represents an empty position. The clenching of the right hand represents a filled up position and the clenching of the left hand represents an empty position. The **_kinesthetic_** representation for the answer which corresponds to the first picture is the clenching of the left hand thrice and right hand. The kinesthetic representation for the second picture is the clenching of the right hand and left hand thrice. The kinesthetic representation for the third picture is the clenching of the left hand twice, right hand, and left hand.

BLUE LESSONS, LESSON 2, Figure 9

In Figure 10 we have a **_visual_** display of two pictures with four positions. Positions one and four are filled up with symbols but positions two and three are empty. The **_audio_** representation of this figure is **knock, double knock, double knock, and knock.**

Figure 9

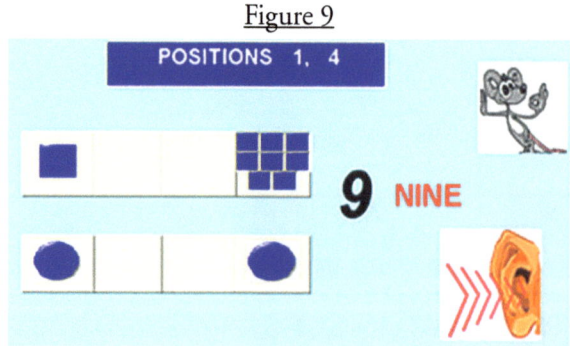

The pictures of boxes correspond to the mathematical value of number nine.

The **_audio_** signal of knock represents the filled up position and double knock represents an empty position. In our example knock, double knock, double knock, and knock correspond to both pictures.

The **_visual_** display of the first picture of boxes has a square symbol in the first place and in the fourth place, but the second place and third place both have empty spaces. There is a circle in the first and second positions of the second picture. The different symbols in the first and fourth positions of the pictures do not change the mathematical representation of both configurations. The shape of the symbols also does not have any effect on the

36

mathematical meaning. The symbols exist just to show that positions are already filled up. The mathematical value of the first configuration as well as the second is equal to nine.

The **kinesthetic** representation for the knock is the clenching of the right hand and for double knock is the tightening of the left hand into a fist. The filled up position is represented by the clenching of the right hand and an empty position represented by the clenching of the left hand. The **kinesthetic** representation for the first and second configurations of boxes is the clenching of the right hand once, left hand twice, and then the right hand once.

BLUE LESSONS, LESSON 2, Figure 10

In Figure 10 we have the **visual** display of two pictures with four positions each. Positions two and four are filled up with symbols. Positions one and three are empty. The **audio** representation of those figures is **double knock, knock, double knock and knock**.

<u>Figure 10</u>

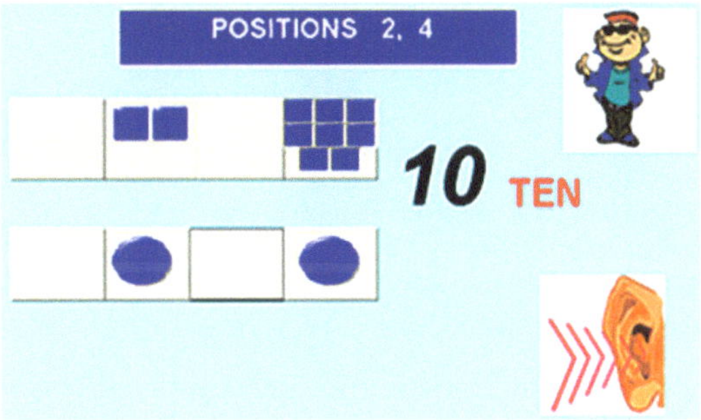

The pictures of boxes correspond to the mathematical value of number ten.

The **audio** signal of knock represents the filled up position and double knock represents an empty position. In our example double knock, knock, double knock, and knock correspond to both pictures. The **video** display of the first picture of boxes has square symbols in the second place and fourth place. First place and third place have empty spaces. In the second and third position of the second picture we see a circle. In the first and second positions we have empty spaces. The shape of the symbols does not affect the mathematical meaning. The symbols exist just to show that positions are already filled up. The mathematical value of the first configuration as well as the second is equal to ten.

The **kinesthetic** representation of the knock is the clenching of the right hand and for double knock is the tightening of the left hand into a fist. The filled up position is represented by the clenching of the right hand and the empty position represented by the clenching of the left hand. The **kinesthetic** representation for the first and second configurations of boxes is the clenching of the left, right, left and right hands.

BLUE LESSONS, LESSON 2, Figure 11

In Figure 11 we have a *__visual__* display of the two pictures with four positions. The positions one, two and four are filled up with symbols but position three is empty. The *__audio__* representation of those figures is **knock, knock, double knock and knock.**

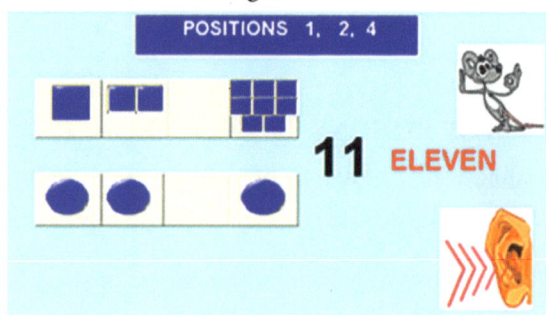

Figure 11

The pictures of boxes correspond to the mathematical value of eleven.

In our example the *__audio__* signals of knock and double knock correspond to both pictures.

The *__visual__* display of the first picture of boxes has a square symbol in the first, second and fourth places, and empty space in the second place. In the first, second and fourth positions of the second picture we see a circle. The different symbols in the first, second and fourth positions of the pictures do not change the mathematical representation of both configurations. The shape of the symbols also does not have any effect on the mathematical meaning. The symbols exist just to show that positions are already filled up. The mathematical value of the first and second configurations is equal to eleven.

The *__kinesthetic__* representation of the knock is the clenching of the right hand and for double knock is the tightening of the left hand into a fist. The filled up position is represented by the clenching of the right hand and the empty position by the clenching of the left hand. The *__kinesthetic__* representation for the first and second configurations of boxes is the clenching of the right hand twice, left once and the then the right hand one last time.

BLUE LESSONS, LESSON 2, Figure 12

In Figure 12, we have a *__visual__* display of two pictures containing four positions each. Positions three and four are filled up with symbols, but the first and second positions are empty.

The *__audio__* representation of this figure is **double knock, double knock, knock, and knock.**

<u>Figure 12</u>

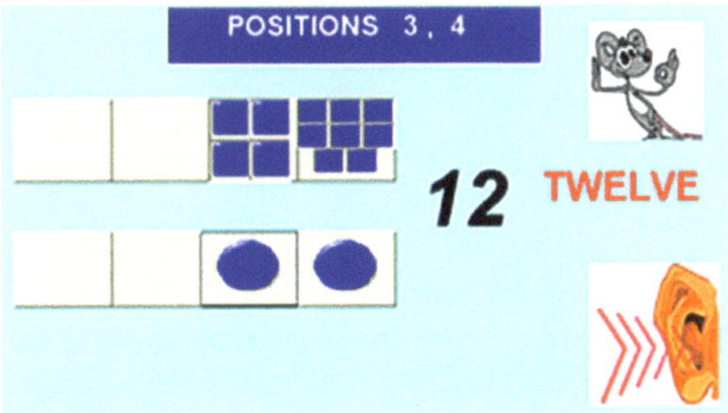

POSITIONS 3, 4

12 TWELVE

The pictures of boxes correspond to the mathematical value of number twelve.

The **audio** signal of knock represents the filled up position and double knock represents an empty position. In our example double knock, double knock, knock and knock correspond to both pictures. The **visual** display of the first picture of boxes has a square symbol in the third and fourth places but empty spaces in the first and second place. In the third and fourth positions of the second picture, we see a circle. The different symbols in the individual positions do not change the mathematical representation of both configurations. The symbols exist just to show that the positions are already filled up. The mathematical value of the first configuration as well as the second is equal to twelve.

The **kinesthetic** representation of the knock is the clenching of the right hand and for double knock is the tightening of the left hand into a fist. The filled up position is represented by the clenching of the right hand and the empty position represented by the clenching of the left hand. The **kinesthetic** representation for the first and second configurations of boxes is the clenching of the left hand twice, then the right hand twice.

BLUE LESSONS, LESSON 2, Figure 13

In Figure 13, we have a **visual** display of two pictures with four positions in each. Positions one, three, and four are filled with symbols and the second position is empty.

The **audio** representation of those figures is **knock, double knock, knock and knock**.

<u>Figure 13</u>

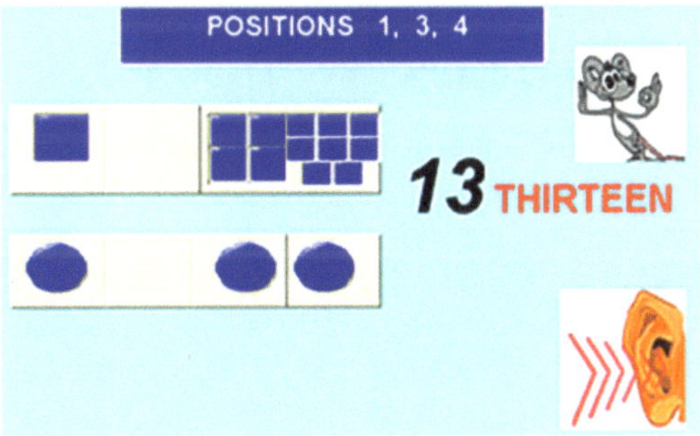

POSITIONS 1, 3, 4

13 THIRTEEN

The pictures of boxes correspond to the mathematical value of number thirteen.

The **audio** signal of knock represents the filled position and the double knock represents the empty position. In our example knock, double knock, knock, and knock correspond to both pictures.

The **visual** display of the first picture of boxes has a square symbol in the first, third and fourth places, but there is empty space in the second place. In the first, third and fourth positions of the second picture we see circles. The mathematical value of the both the first and second configurations is equal to thirteen.

The **kinesthetic** representation of a knock is the clenching of the right hand and for a double knock is the tightening of the left hand into a fist. The **kinesthetic** representation for the first and second configurations of boxes is the clenching of the right, left, and the right twice.

BLUE LESSONS, LESSON 2, Figure 14

In Figure 14, we have a **visual** display of two pictures with four positions each. Position one is empty and the other three positions are filled up with symbols.

The **audio** representation of this figure is **double knock, knock, knock, and knock**.

Figure 14

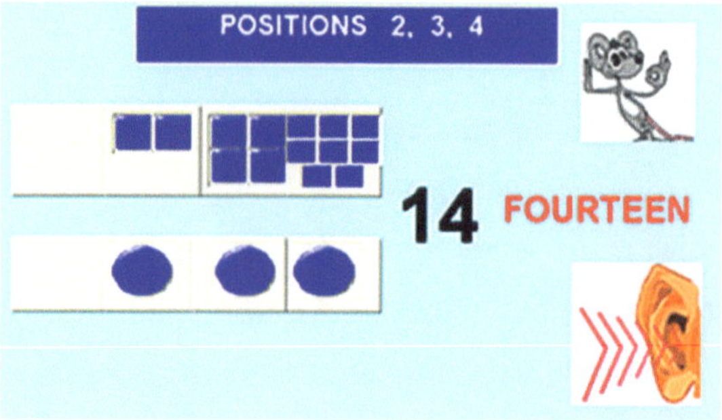

In the pictures above the **audio** signal of knock represents the filled up position and double knock represents an empty position. In our example, double knock, knock, knock, and knock correspond to both pictures.

The **video** display of the first picture of boxes has a square symbol in the second, third, forth place and empty space in the first. In the second, third and forth position of the second picture we have a circle. The symbols and shapes do not change the mathematical representation of both configurations. The symbols are there just to illustrate that positions are already filled up. The mathematical value of the first and second configurations is equal to fourteen.

A filled up position is represented by the clenching of the right hand and an empty position represented by the clenching of the left hand. In conclusion, the **kinesthetic** representation for the first and second configurations of boxes is the clenching of the left hand once and then the right hand three times.

BLUE LESSONS, Figure 15

In Figure 15, in a **visual** display of both pictures we have four positions on each picture. All four positions are filled up with symbols.

The **audio** representation of this figure is **knock, knock, knock and knock**.

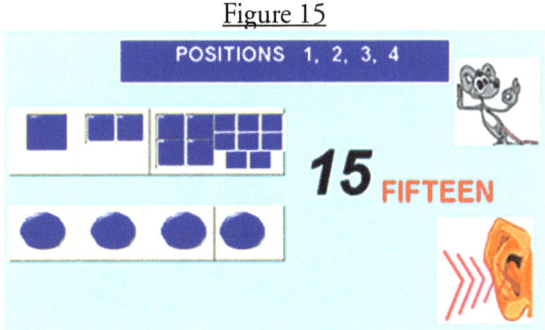

Figure 15

The **audio** signal of knock represents a filled up position. In our example we have four knocks that represent both pictures. In the **video** display of the first picture of boxes, we have a square symbol in all four places. Similarly, we have all places filled up in the second picture, but this time with a circle instead of a square. The symbols are there to indicate that the positions are already filled up. The mathematical value of the first and second configurations is equal to fifteen.

The filled up position is represented by the clenching of the right hand and the empty position is represented by the clenching of the left hand.

The **kinesthetic** representation for the first and second configurations of boxes is the clenching of the right hand four times.

BLUE LESSONS, Figure 16

In Figure 16, in a **visual** display of both pictures we have five positions in each picture. Position five is filled up with symbols and first four positions are empty.

The **audio** representation of this figure is **double knock, double knock, double knock, double knock and knock.**

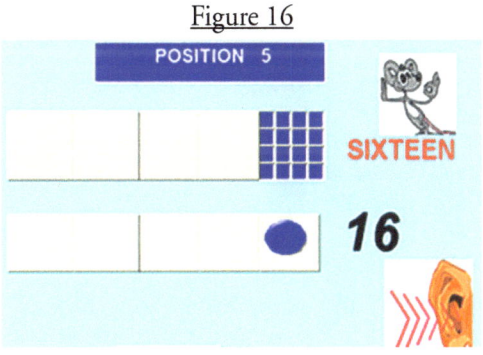

Figure 16

In the first picture of boxes we see square symbols in the fifth place and empty spaces before it. In the fifth position of the second picture we have a circle and empty spaces in the first four positions. The mathematical value of both configurations is equal to sixteen. A filled up position is represented by the clenching of the right hand. An empty position is represented by the clenching of the left hand.

The **kinesthetic** representation for the first and second configurations of boxes is clenching of the left hand four times and then the right hand once.

BLUE LESSONS, Exercise, Figure 9

In Figure 9, we have three *visual* combinations that are filled up with symbols or empty positions. The *audio* representation of one of the pictures below is **knock, double knock, double knock and knock.**

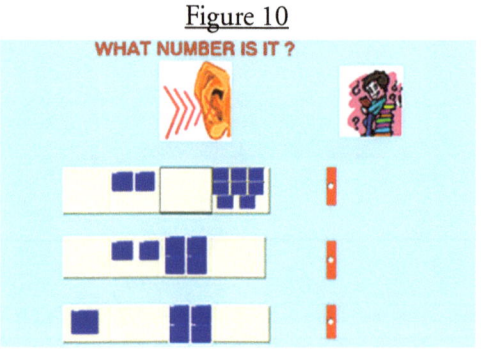

Figure 9

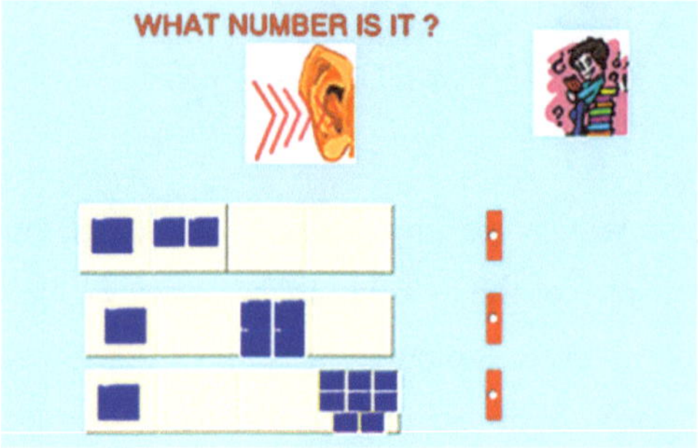

A knock represents a filled up position and a double knock represents an empty position. The clenching of the right hand represents a filled up position and the clenching of the left hand represents an empty position. The *kinesthetic* representation for the answer which corresponds to the third picture is the clenching of the right hand, left hand twice, and right hand. The kinesthetic representation for the first picture is the clenching of the right hand twice and left hand twice. The kinesthetic representation for the second picture is the clenching of the right hand, left hand, right hand, and left hand.

BLUE LESSONS, EXERCISE, Figure 10

In Figure 10, we have three *visual* combinations that are filled up with symbols or empty positions. The *audio* representation of one of the pictures below is **double knock, knock, double knock, and knock.**

Figure 10

A knock represents a filled up position and a double knock represents an empty position. The clenching of the right hand represents a filled up position and the clenching of the left hand represents an empty position. The *kinesthetic* representation for the answer which corresponds to the first picture is the clenching of the left hand, right hand, left hand, and right hand. The kinesthetic representation for the second picture is the clenching of the left hand, right hand twice, and left hand. The kinesthetic representation for the third picture is the clenching of the right hand, left hand, right hand, and left hand.

BLUE LESSONS, EXERCISE, Figure 11

In Figure 11 we have three **_visual_** combinations that are filled up with symbols or empty positions. The **_audio_** representation of one of the pictures below is **knock, knock, double knock, and knock**

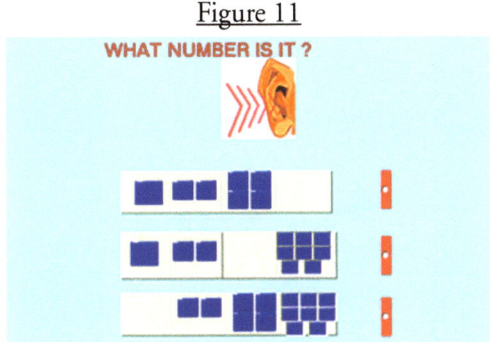

Figure 11

A knock represents a filled up position and a double knock represents an empty position. The clenching of the right hand represents a filled up position and the clenching of the left hand represents an empty position. The **_kinesthetic_** representation for the answer which corresponds to the second picture is the clenching of the right hand twice, left hand, and right hand. The kinesthetic representation for the first picture is the clenching right hand thrice and left hand. The kinesthetic representation for the third picture is the clenching of the left hand and right hand thrice.

BLUE LESSONS, EXERCISE, Figure 12

In Figure 12 we have three **_visual_** combinations that are filled up with symbols or empty positions. The **_audio_** representation of one of the pictures below is **double knock, double knock, knock, and knock**.

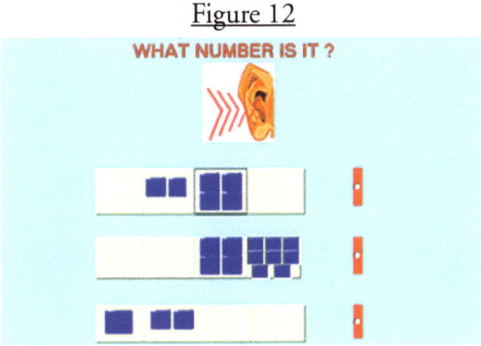

Figure 12

A knock represents a filled up position and a double knock represents an empty position. The clenching of the right hand represents a filled up position and the clenching of the left an empty position. The **_kinesthetic_** representation for the answer corresponding to the second picture is the clenching of the left hand twice and right hand twice. The kinesthetic representation for the first picture is the clenching of the left hand, right hand twice, and left hand. The kinesthetic representation for the third picture is the clenching of the right hand twice and left hand twice.

BLUE LESSONS, EXERCISE, Figure 13

In Figure 13, we have three *visual* combinations that are filled up with symbols or empty positions. The *audio* representation of one of the pictures below is **knock, double knock, knock, and knock**.

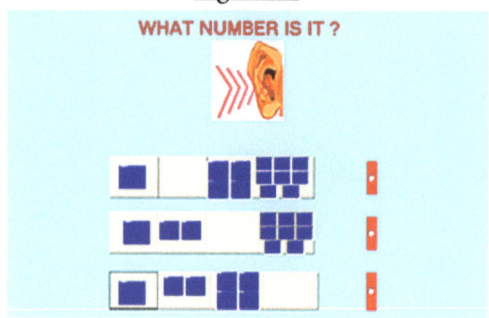

Figure 13

A knock represents a filled up position and a double knock represents an empty position. The clenching of the right hand represents a filled up position and the clenching of the left hand represents an empty position. The *kinesthetic* representation for the answer which corresponds to the first picture is the clenching of the right hand, left hand, and right hand twice. The kinesthetic representation for the second picture is the clenching of the right hand twice, left hand, and right hand. The kinesthetic representation for the third picture is the clenching of the right hand three times and left hand once.

MATHEMATICS
BLUE LESSONS, EXERCISE, Figure 14

In Figure 14, we have three *visual* combinations that are filled up with symbols or empty positions. The *audio* representation of one of the pictures below is **double knock, knock, knock, and knock**.

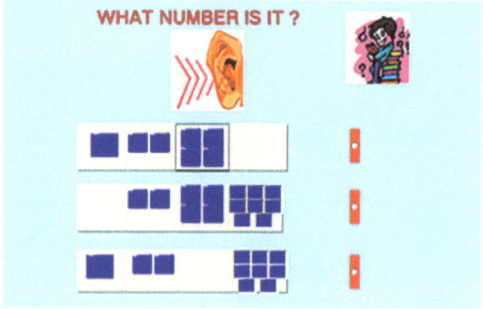

Figure 14

A knock represents a filled up position and a double knock represents an empty position. The clenching of the right hand represents a filled up position and the clenching of the left hand represents an empty position. The *kinesthetic* representation for the answer which corresponds to the second picture is the clenching of the left hand, followed by the right hand thrice. The kinesthetic representation for the first picture is the clenching of the right hand thrice and left hand. The kinesthetic representation for the third picture is the clenching of the right hand twice, left hand, and right hand.

BLUE LESSONS, EXERCISE, Figure 15

In Figure 15, we have three <u>*visual*</u> combinations that are filled with symbols or empty positions. The <u>*audio*</u> representation of one of the pictures below is **knock, knock, knock, and knock**.

Figure 15

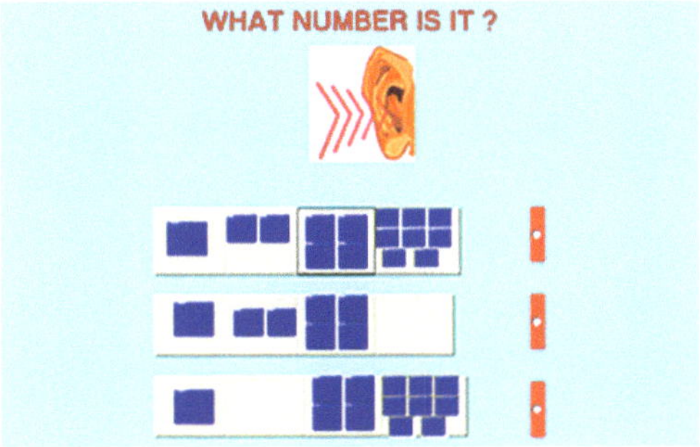

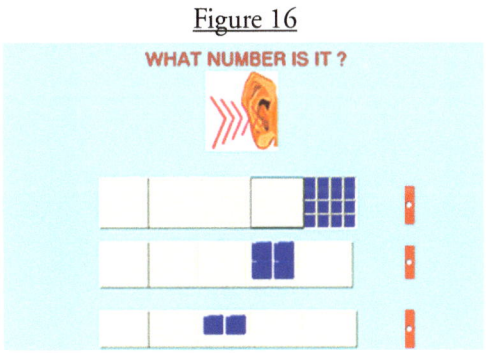

A knock represents a filled position and a double knock represents an empty position. The clenching of the right hand represents a filled position and the clenching of the left hand represents an empty position. The <u>*kinesthetic*</u> representation for the answer which corresponds to the first picture is the clenching of right hand four times. The kinesthetic representation for the second picture is the clenching of the right hand thrice and left hand. The kinesthetic representation for the third picture is the clenching of the right hand, left hand, and right hand twice.

BLUE LESSONS, EXERCISE, Figure 16

In Figure 16 we have three <u>*visual*</u> combinations that are filled up with symbols or empty positions. The <u>*audio*</u> representation of one of the pictures below is **double knock, double knock, double knock, double knock and knock**.

Figure 16

A knock represents a filled up position and a double knock represents an empty position. The clenching of the right hand represents a filled up position and the clenching of the left hand represents an empty position. The <u>*kinesthetic*</u> representation for the answer which corresponds to the first picture is the clenching of the left hand four times and right hand. The kinesthetic representation for the second picture is the clenching of the left hand thrice, right hand, and left hand. The kinesthetic representation for the third picture is the clenching of the left hand twice, right hand, and left hand twice.

BLUE LESSONS, LESSON, Figure 17

In Figure 17, in a ***visual*** display both pictures have five positions, where position one and five are filled up with symbols, and positions two, three and four are empty.

The ***audio*** representation of this figure is a **knock, double knock, double knock, double knock and knock.**

Figure 17

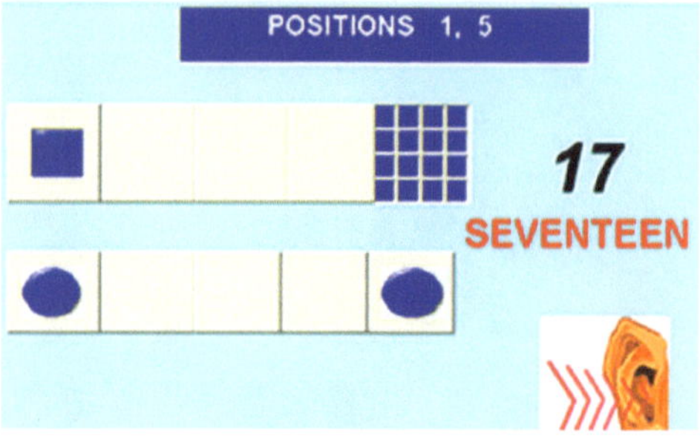

From the diagram we have the **visual** representation of a filled up position represented by a knock and the empty position represented by a double knock. The corresponding **audio** signals are knock, three double knocks and one single knock. In the first picture of boxes there are square symbols in the first and fifth places. In the same positions of the second picture, there are circles. The different symbols and shapes in both pictures do not change the mathematical representation of both configurations. The mathematical value of both configurations is equal to seventeen.

A filled up position is represented by the clenching of the right hand. An empty position is represented by the clenching of the left hand. The ***kinesthetic*** representation for the first and second configurations of boxes is the clenching of the right once, left hand three times and then the right hand once, signifying that our mathematical value is equal to seventeen.

BLUE LESSONS, LESSON, Figure 18

In Figure 18, in a ***visual*** display both pictures have five positions, where positions two and five are filled with symbols, and positions one, three, and four are empty.

The ***audio*** representation of this figure is a **double knock, knock, double knock, double knock and knock.**

Figure 18

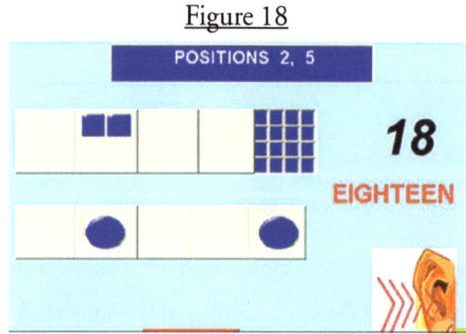

In the first picture of boxes we see square symbols in the second and fifth places. In the next picture we have circles filling up the second and fifth positions. The different symbols and shapes in both pictures do not change the mathematical representation of both configurations. The mathematical value of both configurations is equal to eighteen.

The ***kinesthetic*** representation for the first and second configurations of boxes is the clenching of the left, right, left twice and then the right hand once.

BLUE LESSONS, LESSON, Figure 19

In Figure 19, in both *<u>visual</u>* pictures we have five positions, where positions one, two and five are filled with symbols, and positions three to four are empty.

The *<u>audio</u>* representation of this figure is **knock, knock, double knock, double knock and knock**

Figure 19

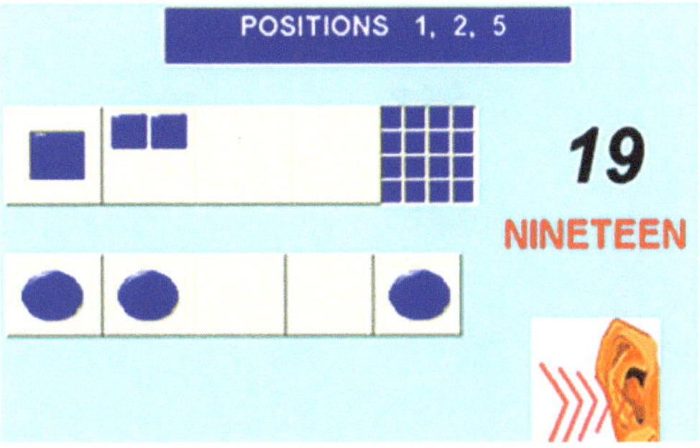

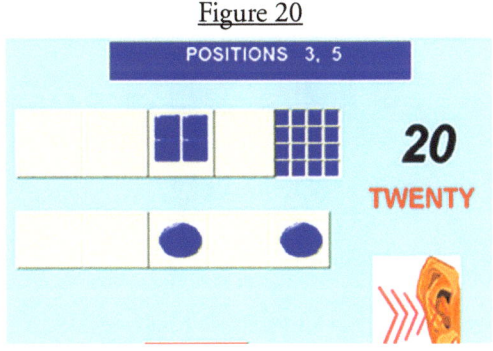

In the first picture of boxes we see square symbols in the first, second and fifth places. In the second picture the first, second and fifth positions are filled with circles. The different symbols and shapes in the pictures do not change the mathematical representation of both configurations. The mathematical value of both configurations is equal to nineteen.

The *<u>kinesthetic</u>* representation for the first and second configurations of boxes is the clenching of the right hand twice, left twice and then the right hand once.

MATHEMATICS
BLUE LESSONS, LESSON, Figure 20

In Figure 20, in both *<u>visual</u>* pictures we have five positions, where positions three and five are filled with symbols, and positions one, two, and four are empty.

The *<u>audio</u>* representation of this figure is **double knock, double knock, knock, double knock and one single knock**.

Figure 20

In the first picture of boxes we see square symbols in the third and fifth place. In the second picture the third and fifth positions are filled with circles. The different symbols and shapes in the pictures do not change the mathematical representation of both configurations. As a result, the mathematical value of both configurations is equal to twenty.

The *<u>kinesthetic</u>* representation for the first and second configurations of boxes is the clenching of the left twice, right once, left once and then the right hand once.

BLUE LESSONS, LESSON, Figure 21

In Figure 21, in both *visual* pictures we have five positions, where positions one, three and five are filled with symbols. In positions two and four we have empty spaces.

In the *audio* representation of both figures we have a **knock, double knock, knock, double knock and knock**.

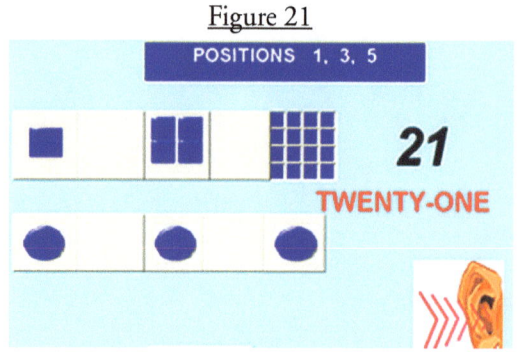

Figure 21

In the first picture of boxes we see square symbols in the first, third and fifth places. In the second picture positions three and five are all filled with circles. The different symbols and shapes in the pictures do not change the mathematical representation of both configurations. As a result the mathematical value of both configurations is equal to twenty one.

The *kinesthetic* representation for the first and second configurations of boxes is the clenching of the right, left, right, left and right hand once.

BLUE LESSONS, LESSON 3, Figure 22

In Figure 22, in both *visual* pictures we have five positions, where positions two, In the first picture of boxes we see square symbols in the second, third and

audio representation of both figures is **double knock, knock, knock, double knock and single knock**.

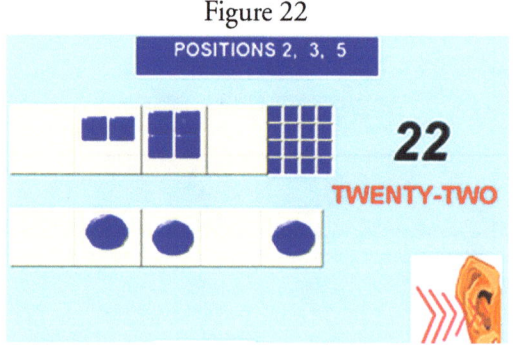

Figure 22

In the second pictures positions two, three and five are filled with circles. The different symbols and shapes in the pictures do not change the mathematical representation of both configurations. The mathematical value of both configurations is equal to twenty two.

The *kinesthetic* representation for the first and second configurations of the boxes is the clenching of the left, right twice, left and right hand once.

BLUE LESSONS, LESSON, Figure 23

In Figure 23, in both **_visual_** representations we have five positions, where positions one, two, three and five are filled with symbols. In position four we have an empty space.

In the **_audio_** representation of both figures we have a **knock, knock knock, double knock, and knock**.

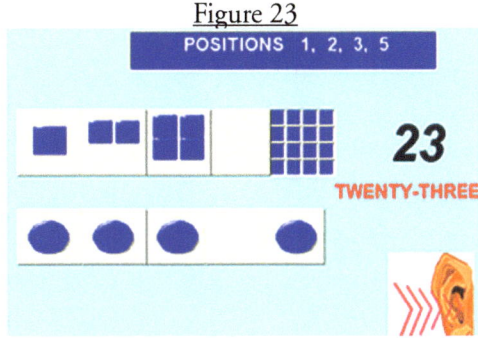

Figure 23

In the first picture of boxes we see square symbols in the first, second, third and fifth places. In the second picture, positions one, two, three and five are filled with circles. The different symbols and shapes in the pictures do not change the mathematical representation of both configurations. The mathematical value of both configurations is equal to twenty three.

The **_kinesthetic_** representation for the first and second configurations of the boxes is the clenching of the right hand three times, left hand once and right hand once.

BLUE LESSONS, LESSON, Figure 24

In Figure 24, in both **_visual_** representations we have five positions, where positions four and five are filled with symbols. Positions one, two, and three have empty spaces in the boxes.

In the **_audio_** representation of both figures we have **three double knocks, and two single knocks**

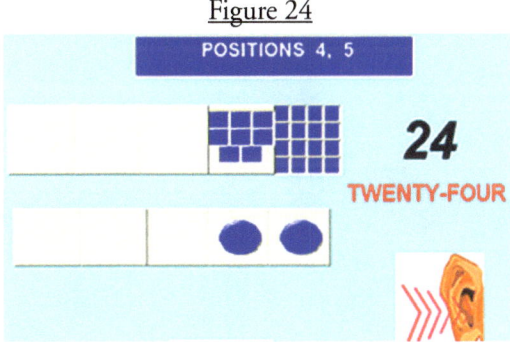

Figure 24

In the first picture of boxes we see square symbols in the fourth and fifth places. In the second picture, positions four and five are filled with circles. The different symbols and shapes in the pictures do not change the mathematical representation of both configurations. The mathematical value of both configurations is equal to twenty four.

The **_kinesthetic_** representation for the first and second configurations of the boxes is the clenching of the left hand three times and right hand twice.

BLUE LESSONS, Exercise, Figure 17

In Figure 17, we have three *visual* combinations that are filled up with symbols or empty positions. The *audio* representation of one of the pictures below is **knock, double knock, double knock, double knock and knock**.

Figure 17

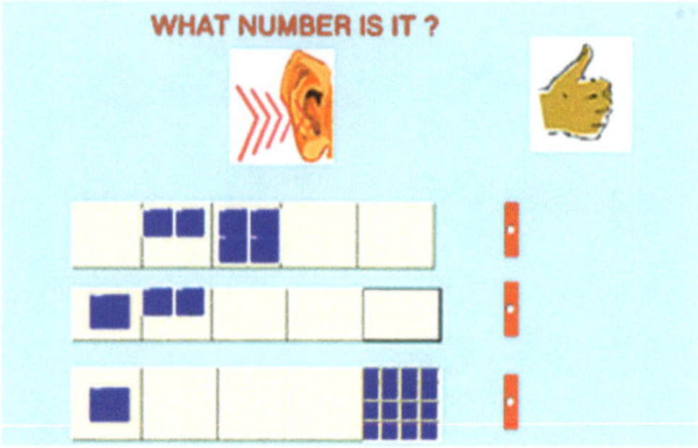

A knock represents a filled up position and a double knock represents an empty position. The clenching of the right hand represents a filled up position and the clenching of the left hand represents an empty position. The *kinesthetic* representation for the answer which corresponds to the third picture is the clenching of right hand, left hand thrice, and right hand. The kinesthetic representation for the second picture is the clenching of the right hand twice and left hand thrice. The kinesthetic representation for the first picture is the clenching of the left hand, right hand twice, and left hand twice.

BLUE LESSONS, Exercise, Figure 18

In Figure 18, we have three *visual* combinations that are filled up with symbols or empty positions. The *audio* representation of one of the pictures below is **double knock, knock, double knock, double knock and knock**.

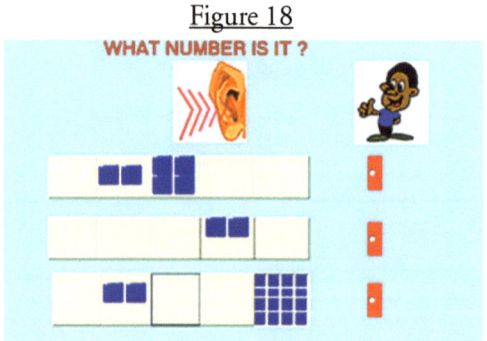

Figure 18

A knock represents a filled up position and a double knock represents an empty position. The clenching of the right hand represents a filled up position and the clenching of the left hand represents an empty position. The *kinesthetic* representation for the answer which corresponds to the third picture is the clenching of the left hand, right hand, left hand twice, and right hand. The kinesthetic representation for the second picture is the clenching of the left hand thrice, right hand, and left hand. The kinesthetic representation for the first picture is the clenching of the left hand, right hand twice, and left hand twice.

BLUE LESSONS, Exercise, Figure 19

In Figure 19, we have three _**visual**_ combinations that are filled up with symbols or empty positions. The _**audio**_ representation of one of the pictures below is **knock, knock, double knock, double knock and knock**.

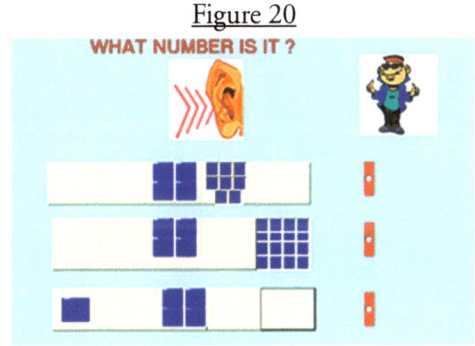

Figure 19

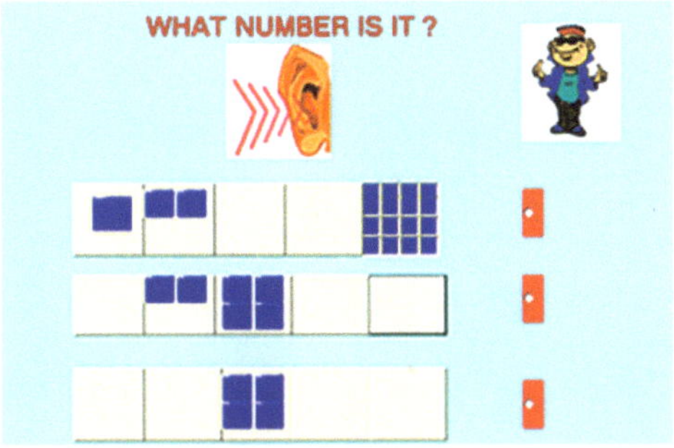

A knock represents a filled up position and a double knock represents an empty position. The clenching of the right hand represents a filled up position and the clenching of the left hand represents an empty position. The _**kinesthetic**_ representation for the answer which corresponds to the first picture is the clenching of the right hand twice, left hand twice, and right hand. The kinesthetic representation for the second picture is the clenching left hand, right hand twice, and left hand twice. The kinesthetic representation for the third picture is the clenching of the left hand twice, right hand, and left hand twice.

BLUE LESSONS, Exercise, Figure 20

In Figure 20, we have three _**visual**_ combinations that are filled up with symbols or empty positions. The _**audio**_ representation of one of the pictures below is **double knock, double knock, knock, double knock, and knock**.

Figure 20

A knock represents a filled up position and a double knock represents an empty position. The clenching of the right hand represents a filled up position and the clenching of the left hand represents an empty position. The _**kinesthetic**_ representation for the answer which corresponds to the second picture is the clenching of the left hand twice, right hand, left hand, and right hand. The kinesthetic representation for the first picture is the clenching of the left hand twice, right hand twice, and left hand. The kinesthetic representation for the third picture is the clenching of the right hand, left hand, right hand, and left hand twice.

BLUE LESSONS, EXERCISE 21, Figure 21

In Figure 21, we have three **_visual_** combinations that are filled up with symbols or empty positions. The **_audio_** representation of one of the pictures below is **knock, double knock, knock, double knock, and knock**.

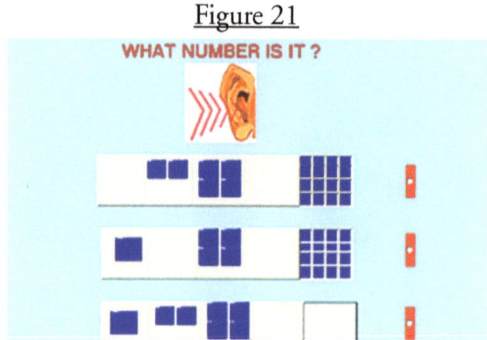

Figure 21

A knock represents a filled up position and a double knock represents an empty position. The clenching of the right hand represents a filled up position and the clenching of the left hand represents an empty position. The **_kinesthetic_** representation for the answer which corresponds to the second picture is the clenching of right hand, left hand, right hand, left hand, and right hand. The kinesthetic representation for the first picture is the clenching of the left hand, right hand twice, left hand, and right hand. The kinesthetic representation for the third picture is the clenching of the right hand thrice and left hand twice.

BLUE LESSONS, EXERCISE 22, Figure 22

In Figure 22, we have three **_visual_** combinations that are filled up with symbols or empty positions. The **_audio_** representation of one of the pictures below is **double knock, knock, knock, double knock, and knock**.

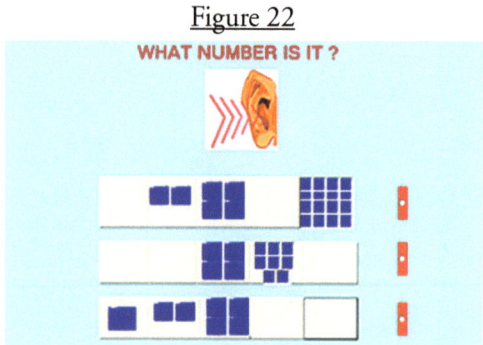

Figure 22

A knock represents a filled up position and a double knock represents an empty position. The clenching of the right hand represents a filled up position and the clenching of the left hand represents an empty position. The **_kinesthetic_** representation for the answer which corresponds to the first picture is the clenching of the left hand, right hand twice, left hand, and right hand. The kinesthetic representation for the second picture is the clenching of the left hand twice, right hand twice, and left hand. The kinesthetic representation for the third picture is the clenching of the right hand thrice and left hand twice.

BLUE LESSONS, EXERCISE 23, Figure 23

In Figure 23, we have three <u>*visual*</u> combinations that are filled up with symbols or empty positions. The <u>*audio*</u> representation of one of the pictures below is **knock, knock, knock, double knock, and knock**.

Figure 23

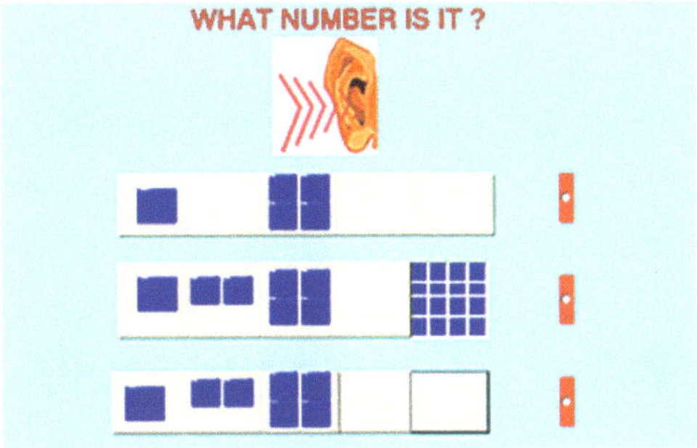

A knock represents a filled up position and a double knock represents an empty position. The clenching of the right hand represents a filled up position and the clenching of the left hand represents an empty position. The <u>*kinesthetic*</u> representation for the answer which corresponds to the second picture is the clenching of right hand thrice, left hand, and right hand. The kinesthetic representation for the first picture is the clenching of the right hand, left hand, right hand, and left hand twice. The kinesthetic representation for the third picture is the clenching of the right hand thrice and left hand twice.

BLUE LESSONS, Figure 24

In Figure 24, we have three <u>*visual*</u> combinations that are filled up with symbols or empty positions. The <u>*audio*</u> representation of one of the pictures below is **double knock, double knock, double knock, knock, and knock**.

Figure 24

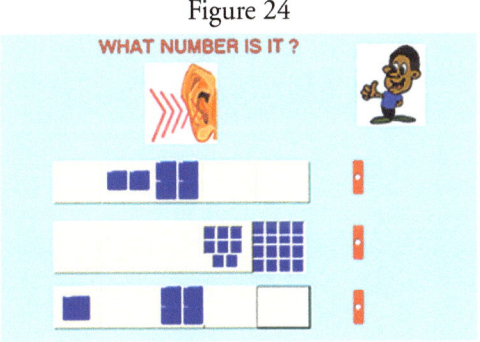

A knock represents a filled up position and a double knock represents an empty position. The clenching of the right hand represents a filled up position and the clenching of the left hand represents an empty position. The <u>*kinesthetic*</u> representation for the answer which corresponds to the second picture is the clenching of the left hand thrice and right hand twice. The kinesthetic representation for the first picture is the clenching of the left hand, right hand twice, and left hand twice. The kinesthetic representation for the third picture is the clenching of the right hand, left hand, right hand, and left hand twice.

BLUE LESSONS, LESSON 4, Figure 25

In Figure 25, in a ***visual*** display in both pictures we have five positions each, where positions one, four and five are filled with symbols. In positions two and three, we have empty spaces in the boxes.

In the **audio** representation of both figures we have a **knock, double knock, double knock, knock and knock**.

Figure 25

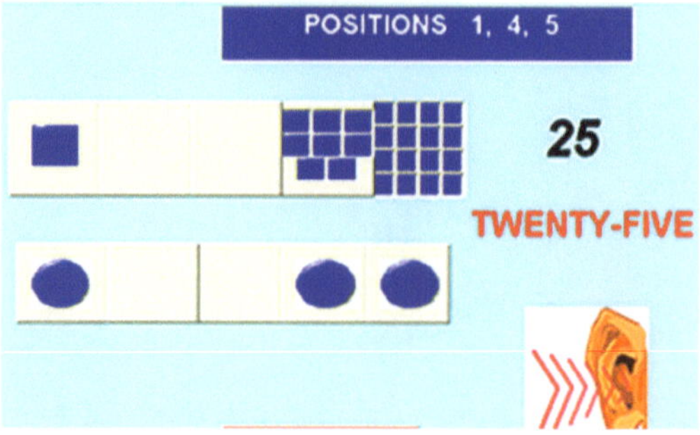

In the first picture of boxes we see square symbols in the first, fourth and fifth places. In the second picture, positions one, four and five are filled with circles. The different symbols and shapes in the pictures do not change the mathematical representation of both configurations. The mathematical value of both configurations is equal to twenty five.

The **kinesthetic** representation for the first and second configurations of boxes is the clenching of the right hand once, left twice and right hand twice.

BLUE LESSONS, LESSON 4, Figure 26

In Figure 26, we have a **visual** display of two pictures. In both pictures we have five positions, where positions two, four and five are filled up with symbols, and positions one and three are empty.

In the **audio** representation of both figures we have a **double knock, knock, double knock, knock and knock**.

Figure 26

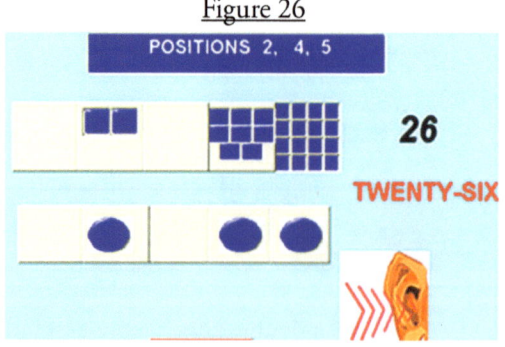

While the first picture has its positions filled with twenty six squares, the same positions in the second picture are filled with symbols. The different symbols and shapes in the pictures do not change the mathematical representation of both configurations, which is equal to twenty six.

The **kinesthetic** representation for the first and second configurations of boxes is *the clenching of the left, right, left and right hand twice.*

BLUE LESSONS, LESSON 4, Figure 27

In Figure 27, we have a **_visual_** display of two pictures. In both pictures we have five positions, where positions one two, four and five are filled with symbols, and position three is empty.

In the **audio** representation of both figures we have a **knock, knock, double knock, knock and knock.**

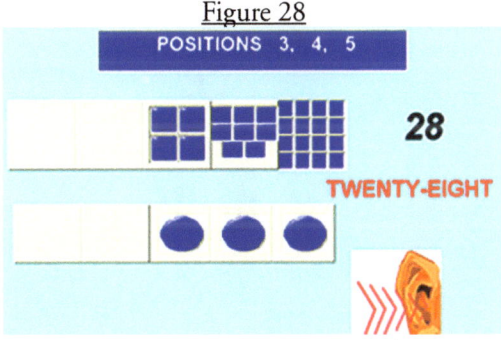

Figure 27

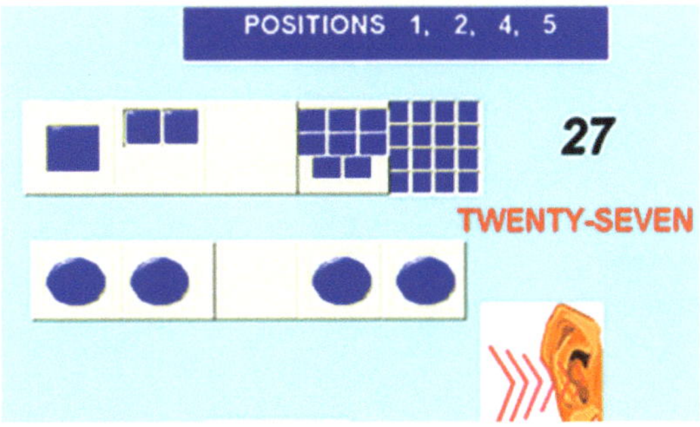

While the first picture has its positions filled with squares, the second picture has the same positions filled with circles. The different symbols and shapes in the pictures do not change the mathematical representation of both configurations. The mathematical value of both configurations is equal to twenty seven.

The **_kinesthetic_** representation for the first and second configurations of boxes is *the clenching of the right twice, left once and right hand twice.*

BLUE LESSONS, LESSON 4, Figure 28

In Figure 28, in a **_visual_** display of the pictures below, positions one and two are empty, while positions three four and five are filled with symbols. In the **_audio_** representation of both figures we have a **double knock, double knock, knock, knock and knock**.

Figure 28

While the first picture has its last three positions filled with square symbols, the same positions in the second picture are filled with circles. The different symbols and shapes in the pictures do not change the mathematical representation of both configurations. The mathematical value of both configurations is equal to twenty eight.

The **_kinesthetic_** representation for the first and second configurations of boxes is *the clenching of the left hand twice and right hand three times.*

BLUE LESSONS, LESSON 4, Figure 29

In Figure 29, in a ***visual*** display of the pictures below, positions one, three, four, and five are filled with symbols, while position two is empty.

In the ***audio*** representation of both figures we have a **knock, double knock, knock, knock and knock**.

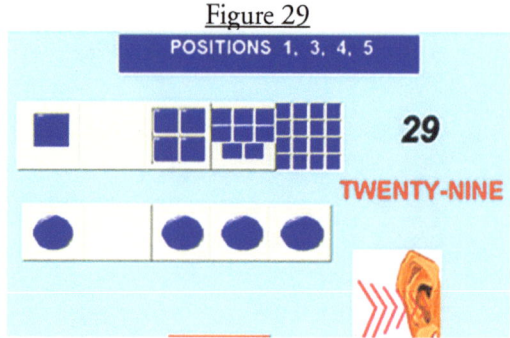

While the first picture has its positions filled with squares, the same positions in the second picture are filled with circles. The different symbols and shapes in the pictures do not change the mathematical representation of both configurations, which is equal to twenty nine.

The ***kinesthetic*** representation for the first and second configurations of boxes is *the clenching of the right hand once, left once and right hand three times.*

BLUE LESSONS, EXERCISE, Figure 25

In Figure 25, we have three ***visual*** combinations that are filled up with symbols or empty positions.

The ***audio*** representation of one of the pictures below is **knock, double knock, double knock, knock, and knock**.

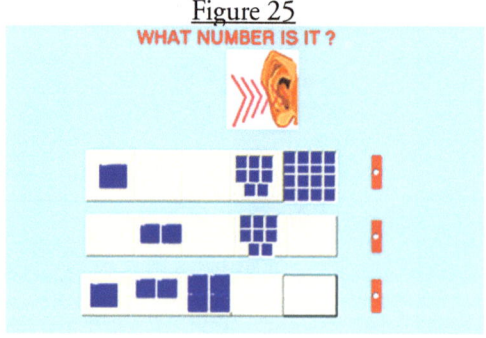

A knock represents a filled up position and a double knock represents an empty position. The clenching of the right hand represents a filled up position and the clenching of the left hand represents an empty position. The ***kinesthetic*** representation for the answer which corresponds to the first picture is the clenching of the right hand, left hand twice, and right hand twice. The kinesthetic representation for the second picture is the clenching of the left hand, right hand, left hand, right hand, and left hand. The kinesthetic representation for the third picture is the clenching of the right hand thrice and left hand twice.

BLUE LESSONS, EXERCISE, Figure 26

In Figure 26, we have three **_visual_** combinations that are filled with symbols or empty positions.

The **_audio_** representation of one of the pictures below is **double knock, knock, double knock, knock, and knock**

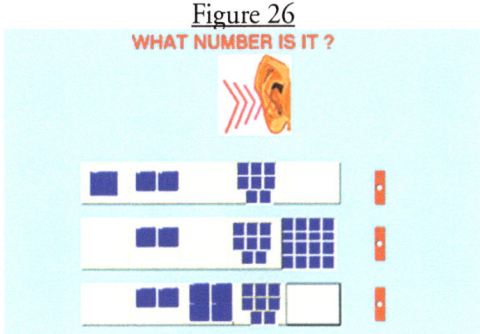

A knock represents a filled up position and a double knock represents an empty position. The clenching of the right hand represents a filled up position and the clenching of the left hand represents an empty position. The **_kinesthetic_** representation for the answer which corresponds to the second picture is the clenching of the left hand, right hand, left hand, and right hand twice. The kinesthetic representation for the first picture is the clenching of the left hand twice, right hand, left hand, and right hand. The kinesthetic representation for the third picture is the clenching of the left hand, right hand thrice, and left hand.

BLUE LESSONS, EXERCISE, Figure 27

In Figure 27, we have three **_visual_** combinations that are filled with symbols or empty positions. The **_audio_** representation of one of the pictures below is **knock, knock, double knock, knock, and knock**.

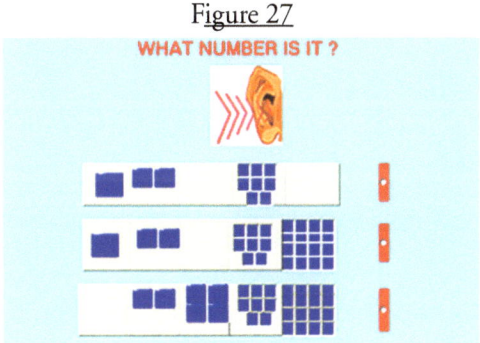

A knock represents a filled up position and a double knock represents an empty position. The clenching of the right hand represents a filled up position and the clenching of the left hand represents an empty position. The **_kinesthetic_** representation for the answer which corresponds to the second picture is the clenching of right hand twice, left hand, and right hand twice. The kinesthetic representation for the first picture is the clenching of the right hand twice, left hand, right hand, and left hand. The kinesthetic representation for the third picture is the clenching of the left hand and right hand four times.

BLUE LESSONS, EXERCISE, Figure 28

In Figure 28, we have three **_visual_** combinations that are filled with symbols or empty positions. The **_audio_** representation of one of the pictures below is **double knock, double knock, knock, knock, and knock**.

Figure 28

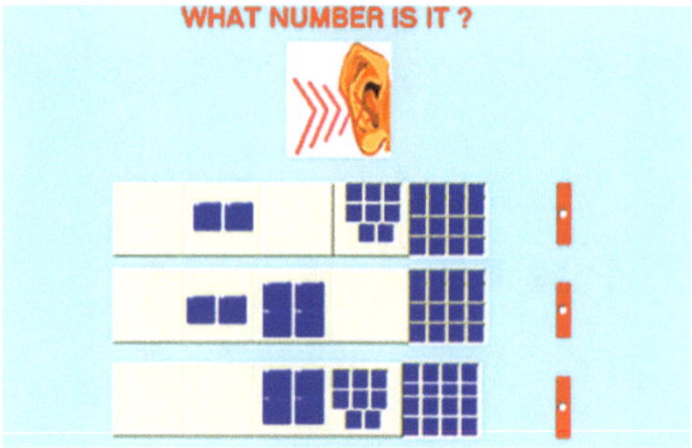

A knock represents a filled up position and a double knock represents an empty position. The clenching of the right hand represents a filled up position and the clenching of the left hand represents an empty position. The **_kinesthetic_** representation for the answer which corresponds to the third picture is the clenching of the left hand twice and right hand thrice. The kinesthetic representation for the first picture is the clenching of the left hand, right hand, left hand, and right hand. The kinesthetic representation for the second picture is the clenching of the left hand, right hand twice, left hand, and right hand.

BLUE LESSONS, EXERCISE, Figure 29

In Figure 29, we have three **_visual_** combinations that are filled with symbols or empty positions. The **_audio_** representation of one of the pictures below is **knock, double knock, knock, knock, and knock**.

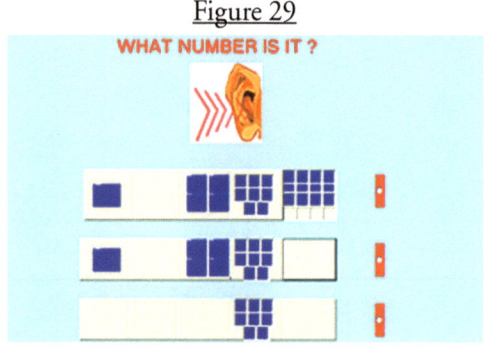

Figure 29

A knock represents a filled up position and a double knock represents an empty position. The clenching of the right hand represents a filled up position and the clenching of the left hand represents an empty position. The **_kinesthetic_** representation for the answer which corresponds to the first picture is the clenching of the right hand, left hand, and right hand thrice. The kinesthetic representation for the second picture is the clenching of the right hand, left hand, right hand twice, and left hand. The kinesthetic representation for the third picture is the clenching of the left hand thrice, right hand, and left hand.

BLUE LESSONS, LESSON, Figure 30

In Figure 30, in both _**visual**_ pictures we have five positions, where positions two through to five are filled with symbols. Position one has an empty space. In the _**audio**_ representation of both figures we have a **double knock, knock, knock, knock and knock**.

Figure 30

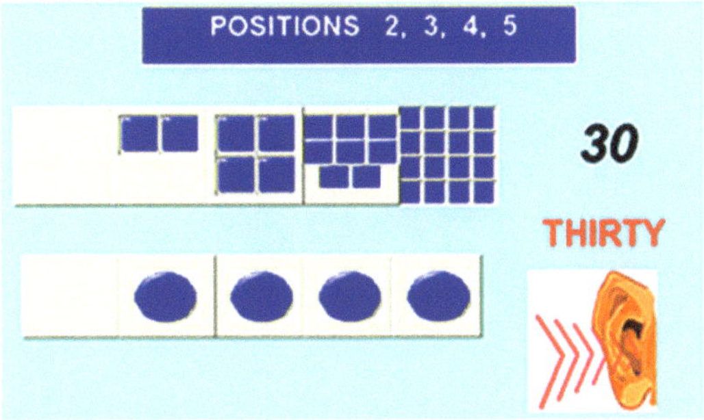

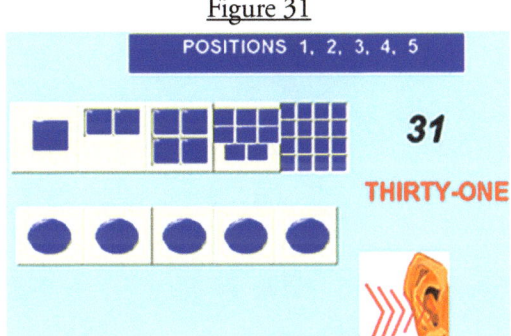

In the first picture of boxes we see square symbols filled in positions two, three, four and five. In the second picture positions two through five are also filled with circles. The different symbols and shapes in the pictures do not change the mathematical representation of both configurations. The mathematical value of both configurations is equal to thirty.

The _**kinesthetic**_ representation for the first and second configurations of the boxes is the clenching of the left hand once and the right hand four times.

BLUE LESSONS, LESSON, Figure 31

In Figure 31, in both _**visual**_ pictures we have five positions, where all positions are filled with symbols.

In the _**audio**_ representation of both figures we have **knock, knock, knock, knock and knock**.

Figure 31

In both pictures of boxes we have all positions filled with both square and circle symbols. The different symbols and shapes in the pictures do not change the mathematical representation of both configurations. The mathematical value of both configurations is equal to thirty one.

The _**kinesthetic**_ representation for the first and second configurations of the boxes is the clenching of the right hand five times.

BLUE LESSONS, EXERCISE 30, Figure 30

In Figure 30, we have three **_visual_** combinations that are filled with symbols or empty positions.

The **_audio_** representation of one of the pictures below is **double knock, knock, knock, knock, and knock**.

Figure 30

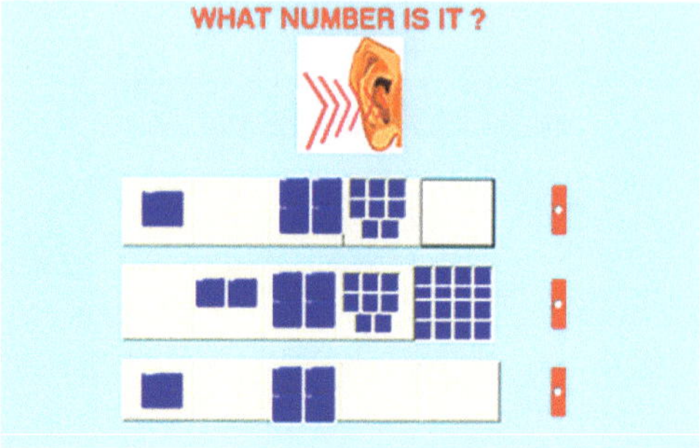

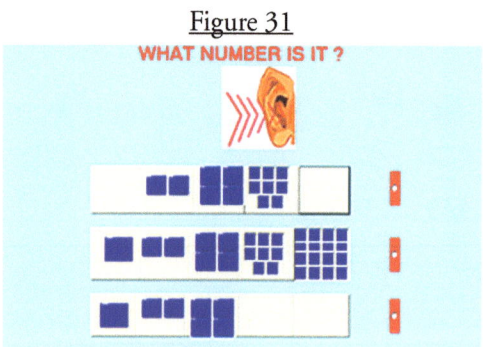

A knock represents a filled position and a double knock represents an empty position. The clenching of the right hand represents a filled position and the clenching of the left hand represents an empty position. The **_kinesthetic_** representation for the answer which corresponds to the second picture is *the clenching of the left hand and right hand four times*. The kinesthetic representation for the first picture is *the clenching of the right hand, left hand, right hand twice, and left hand*. The kinesthetic representation for the third picture is *the clenching of the right hand, left hand, right hand, and left hand twice*.

BLUE LESSONS, EXERCISE, Figure 31

In Figure 31, we have three **_visual_** combinations that are filled with symbols or empty positions.

The **_audio_** representation of one of the pictures below is **knock, knock, knock, knock, and knock**.

Figure 31

A knock represents a filled position and a double knock represents an empty position. The clenching of the right hand represents a filled position and the clenching of the left hand represents an empty position. The **_kinesthetic_** representation for the answer which corresponds to the second picture is *the clenching of the right hand five times*. The kinesthetic representation for the first picture is *the clenching of the left hand, right hand thrice, and left hand*. The kinesthetic representation for the third picture is *the clenching of the right hand thrice and left hand twice*.

INTRODUCTION

TO POSITIONS

INTRODUCTION TO POSITIONS: LESSON 1

In Figure 1 there are two pictures of boxes. There is a combination of positions, filled with symbols or empty spaces. A knock represents a filled position and a double knock represents an empty position. We are balancing our visual and audio reaction on the symbol (knock). The audio representation of one of the pictures below is **knock and double knock**.

<u>Figure 1</u>

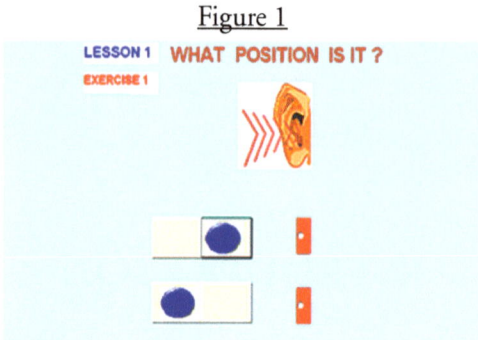

In our example knock and double knock correspond to the second picture. The first drawing of the boxes corresponds to double knock and knock.

The kinesthetic representation involves movement. The method of representation of a knock is clenching of the right fist, and double knock is clenching the left fist. Clenching of the right hand then represents the filled position and left hand clenching represents the empty space. In our example, kinesthetic representation for the answer is *to clench the right hand then the left*. For the first picture the kinesthetic representation is *clenching of the left hand then right hand*.

INTRODUCTION TO POSITIONS: LESSON 2

In Figure 2 we have three combinations of positions, filled with symbols or empty spaces. The audio representation of one of the pictures below is **double knock and knock.**

<u>Figure 2</u>

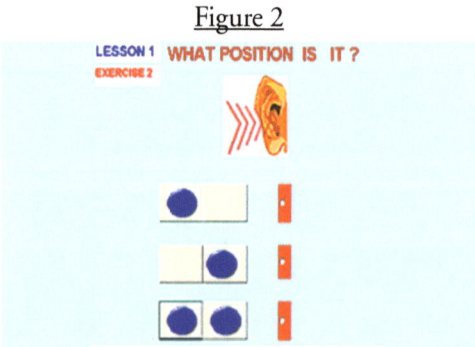

A double knock represents an empty space and a knock represents a filled space. In our example, double knock and knock correspond to the second picture. In accordance with the audio representations, the first picture of boxes corresponds to knock and double knock, and the third represents knock, knock.

The kinesthetic representation of the double knock is clenching of the left hand, and for knock is tightening the right hand into a fist. Clenching of the right hand represents a filled position, and left hand clenching represents an empty position. For the first picture of boxes, kinesthetic representation is clenching of the right then the left hand, and for the third picture kinesthetic representation will be clenching of the right hand twice.

INTRODUCTION TO POSITIONS: LESSON 3

In Figure 3 we have three different combinations of positions, filled with symbols or empty spaces. The audio representation of one of the pictures below is represented by **knock, knock.**

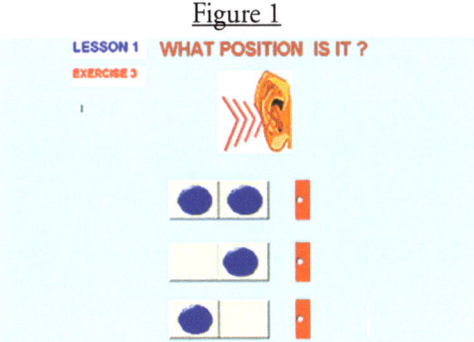

Figure 1

The knock, knock visually represents two filled spaces. In our example knock and knock corresponds to the first picture of boxes. The second picture represents double knock, and knock, and the third picture of boxes corresponds to knock and double knock.

The kinesthetic representation of the answer knock and knock is the *clenching of the right hand twice.* For the second picture of the boxes *clenching of the left hand* represents double knock *and clenching of the right hand* represents knock. A knock and then a double knock represent the third picture. The kinesthetic representation is *clenching of the right and left hand.*

INTRODUCTION TO POSITIONS: LESSON 4

In Figure 4 we have three combinations of filled or empty spaces. The audio representation of one of the pictures below is **knock, double knock, and double knock.**

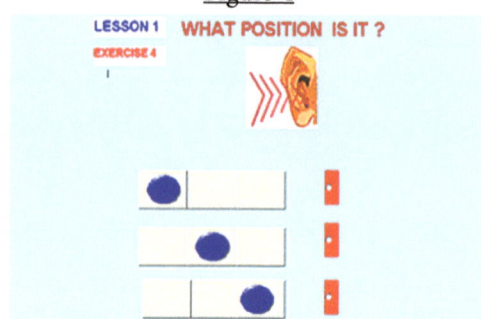

Figure 4

In this figure the first picture of the boxes with the filled space and two empty spaces, is the right answer.

The kinesthetic representation of the answer for knock is *clenching of the right hand, and making a fist with the left hand* <u>two</u> *times* represents the two empty positions.

For the second picture of boxes audio representation is double knock, knock, and double knock. Audio representation for the third picture of boxes is double knock, double knock, and knock.

INTRODUCTION TO POSITIONS: LESSON 5

In Figure 5 we have three combinations of filled or empty spaces. The audio representation of one of the pictures below is **double knock, knock, knock.**

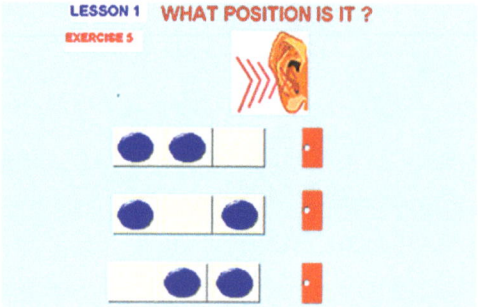

Figure 5

The visual representation of the answer is the third picture, where the first space is empty, and the second and third spaces are filled with a symbol.

The kinesthetic representation of the answer would be *clenching of the left hand once* for the empty position *and the right hand twice* for the second and third filled positions.

INTRODUCTION TO POSITIONS: LESSON 6

In Figure 6 we have three combinations of filled and empty spaces. The audio representation of one of the pictures below is **knock, double knock, knock.**

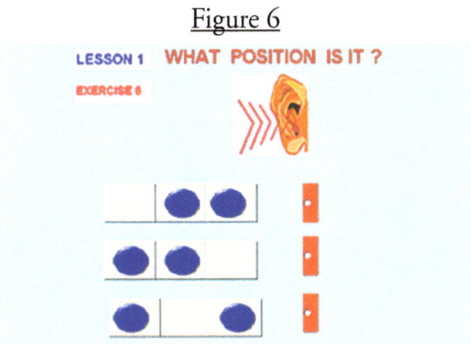

Figure 6

The answer is the third picture of boxes. The visual representation of the answer would be the first position filled with a symbol, the second position empty, and third position filled with a symbol.

The kinesthetic representation of the answer is *clenching of the right hand* for the first position, *clenching of the left* for the second position and *clenching of the right hand* to represent the third position.

INTRODUCTION TO POSITIONS: LESSON 7

In Figure 7 we have three combinations that are filled with symbols or empty spaces. The audio representation of one of the pictures below is **knock, knock, and knock.**

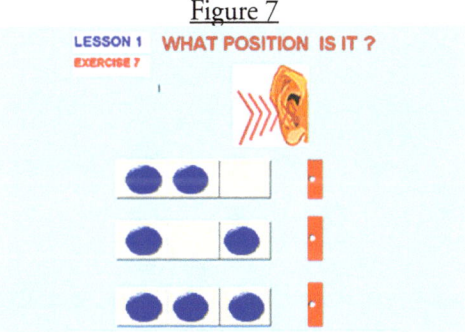

Figure 7

The visual representation of the answer is the third picture of the boxes, where all three spaces are filled with a symbol.

The kinesthetic representation of the answer is *clenching of the right hand three times* in a row to represent the filled positions with symbols.

INTRODUCTION TO POSITIONS: LESSON 8

In Figure 8 we have three combinations of filled or empty spaces. The audio representation of one of the pictures below is **double knock, double knock, double knock, and knock.**

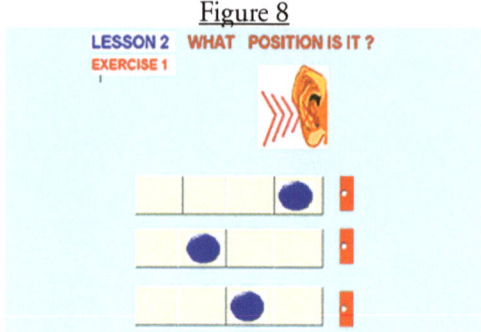

Figure 8

The answer is the first picture of the boxes. The visual representation of the answer has the first three spaces left empty. The fourth position is filled with a symbol.

The kinesthetic representation of the answer is *clenching of the left hand three times*, followed by the *clenching of the right hand once*.

INTRODUCTION TO POSITIONS: LESSON 9

In Figure 9 we have three combinations that are filled with symbols or empty spaces. The audio representation of one of the pictures below is **knock, double knock, double knock, knock.**

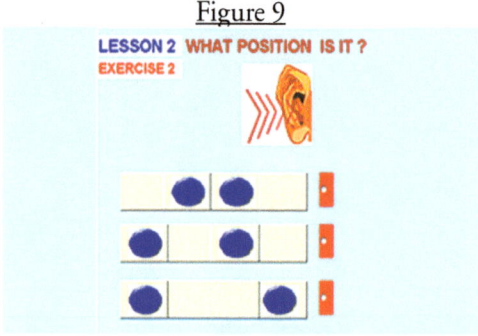

Figure 9

The answer for the audio representations is the third picture of boxes. The visual representation of the answer is a symbol in the first space followed by the second and third spaces being left empty and the fourth space filled with a symbol.

The kinesthetic representation of the answer is *clenching of the right hand* for the first position, followed by the second and third positions being represented by *clenching of the left hand twice and the clenching of the right hand* to represent the symbol in the fourth position.

INTRODUCTION TO POSITIONS: LESSON 10

In Figure 10 we have three combinations that are filled with symbols or empty spaces. The audio representation of one of the pictures below is **double knock, knock, knock, and double knock.**

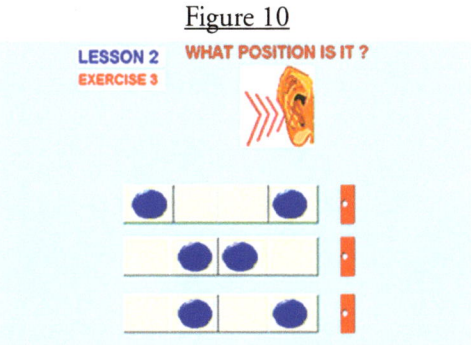

The answer is the second picture of boxes. In the visual representation of the answer, the first space is empty, followed by the second and third spaces filled with symbols and finally the fourth space being empty.

The kinesthetic representation of the answer is the *clenching of the left hand* for the first position, followed by *clenching of the right hand twice* to indicate the presence of symbols in the second and third positions. Finally, *clenching of the left hand* indicates the absence of a symbol in the fourth position.

INTRODUCTION TO POSITIONS: LESSON 11

In Figure 11 we have three combinations that are filled with symbols or empty spaces. The audio representation of one of the pictures below is **knock, knock, double knock, and knock.**

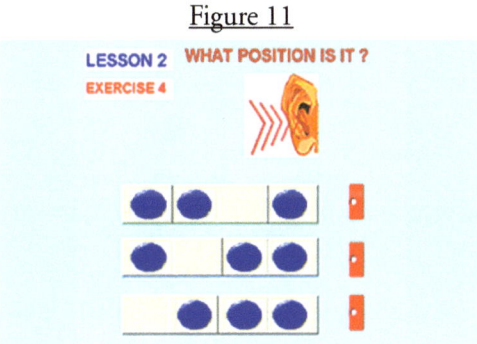

The correct answer in audio representation is the first picture of boxes. In the visual representation of the answer the first and second spaces are filled with a symbol, followed by the third empty space and the fourth space that is filled with a symbol.

The kinesthetic representation of the answer is the *clenching of the right hand twice* for the first and second positions, followed by *clenching of the left hand once* to represent an empty space in the third position. Finally, the *clenching of the right hand* is to represent a symbol in the fourth position.

INTRODUCTION TO POSITIONS: LESSON 12

In Figure 12 we have three combinations that are filled with symbols or empty spaces. The audio representation of one of the pictures below is **double knock, double knock, knock, and knock.**

Figure 12

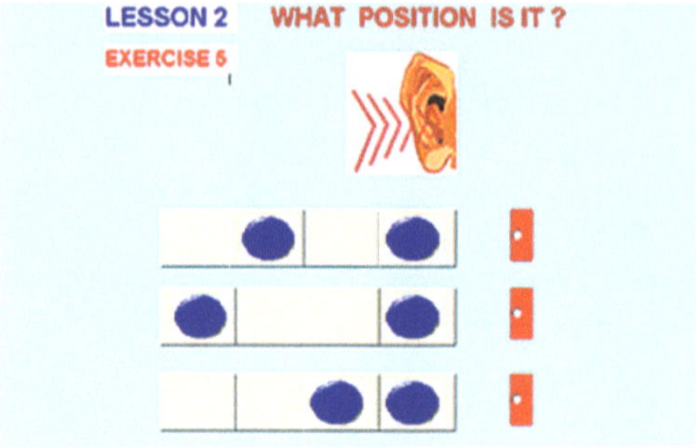

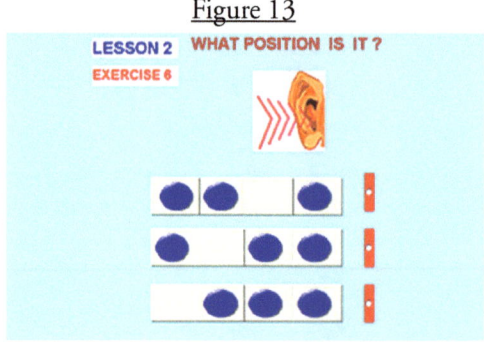

The answer in audio representations is the third picture of boxes. In the visual representation of the answer the first and second squares are empty, followed by third and fourth squares being filled with a symbol.

The kinesthetic representation of the answer is *clenching of the left hand twice* for the first and second positions, followed by *clenching of the right hand twice* to represent the presence of a symbol in the third and fourth positions.

INTRODUCTION TO POSITIONS: LESSON 13

In Figure 13 we have three combinations filled with symbols or empty squares. The audio representation of one of the pictures below is **knock, double knock, knock, and knock.**

Figure 13

The answer for one of the pictures above in audio representations is the second picture of boxes. In the visual representation of the answer the first position contains a symbol, while the second square is empty, followed by a symbol in the third and fourth positions.

The kinesthetic representation of the answer is *clenching of the right hand* for the first position, *followed by clenching the left hand once* to represent a blank space, and the *clenching of the right hand twice* to represent a symbol in the third and fourth positions.

INTRODUCTION TO POSITIONS: LESSON 14

In Figure 14 we have three combinations filled with symbols or empty squares. The audio representation of one of the pictures below is **knock, knock, knock, and double knock.**

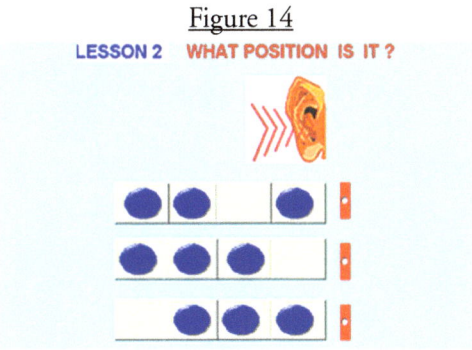

Figure 14

The answer for one of the pictures above in audio representations is the second picture of boxes. In the visual representation of the answer the first, second and third positions are filled with symbols, while the fourth square is empty.

The kinesthetic representation of the answer is the *clenching of the right hand three times* to represent the presence of a symbol in the first, second and third positions, followed by the *clenching of the left hand* to indicate an empty square.

INTRODUCTION TO POSITIONS: LESSON 15

In Figure 15 we have three combinations that are filled with symbols or empty squares. The audio representation of one of the pictures below is **knock, knock, knock, and knock.**

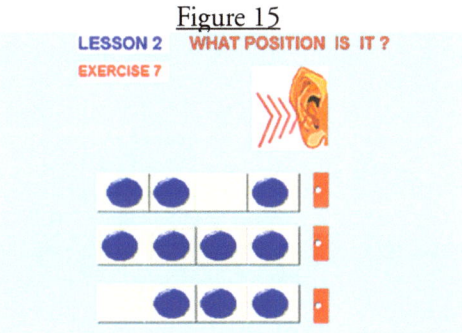

Figure 15

The answer for the picture above in audio representation is the second picture of the boxes. In the visual representation the answer requires all the positions to be filled with a symbol.

The kinesthetic representation of the answer is *clenching of the right hand four times* for the first, second, third and fourth positions to indicate the presence of a symbol.

INTRODUCTION TO POSITIONS: LESSON 16

In Figure 16 we have three combinations that are filled with symbols or empty positions. The audio representation of one of the pictures below is **double knock, knock, double knock, double knock and knock.**

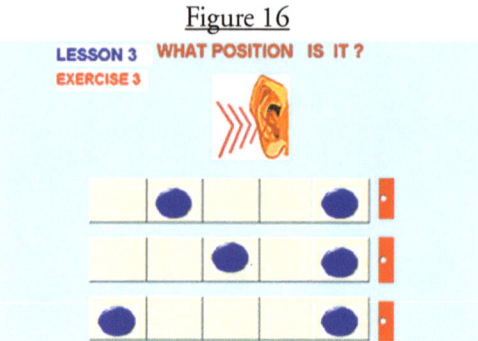

Figure 16

The answer for the assignment above in the audio representation is the first picture of boxes. In the visual representation of the answer the first box is empty, while the second contains a symbol, followed by the third and fourth positions, which are empty, while the fifth square is filled with a symbol.

The kinesthetic representation of the answer is *clenching of the left hand* for the first position, followed by *clenching the right hand* to represent presence of a symbol in the second square. The third and fourth positions are indicated by *clenching of the left hand twice, followed by clenching of the right hand* to indicate the presence of a symbol in the fifth square.

INTRODUCTION TO POSITIONS: LESSON 17

In Figure 17 we have three combinations that are filled up with symbols or empty positions. The audio representation of one of the pictures below is **double knock, knock, double knock, double knock and knock.**

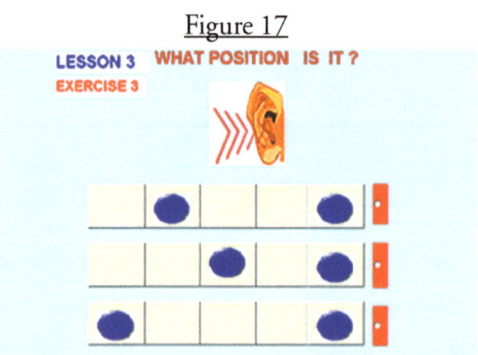

Figure 17

The answer for the assignment above in the audio representations is the first picture of boxes. In the visual representation of the answer the first position is empty and the second is filled with a symbol, followed by the third and fourth positions which are empty, while the fifth box is filled with a symbol.

The kinesthetic representation of the answer is the clenching *of the left hand once* to represent an empty box in the first position, followed by *clenching the right fist* to indicate the presence of a symbol. The third and fourth positions, which are empty, are represented by *clenching the left hand twice*. The *right hand is clenched* to indicate a symbol in the last box.

INTRODUCTION TO POSITIONS: LESSON 18

In Figure 18 we have three combinations that are filled up with symbols or empty positions. The audio representation of one of the pictures below is **knock, double knock, double knock, double knock and knock**.

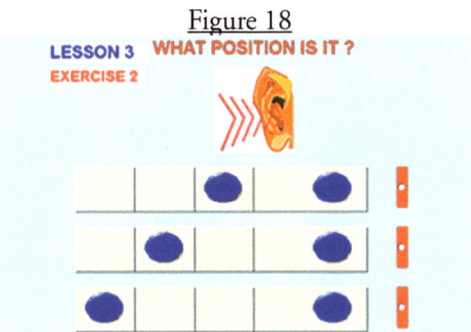

Figure 18

The answer for the audio representations is the third picture of boxes. The visual representation of the answer is for the first position that is filled with a symbol, followed by the second, third and fourth positions being empty, and finally the fifth box containing a symbol.

The kinesthetic representation of the answer is *clenching of the right hand* for the first position, followed by the second third and fourth positions being represented by *clenching of the left hand three times and finally clenching of the right hand* to represent a symbol in the fifth position.

INTRODUCTION TO POSITIONS: LESSON 19

In Figure 19 we have three combinations that contain symbols or empty boxes. The audio representation of one of the pictures below is **knock, knock, double knock, double knock and knock**.

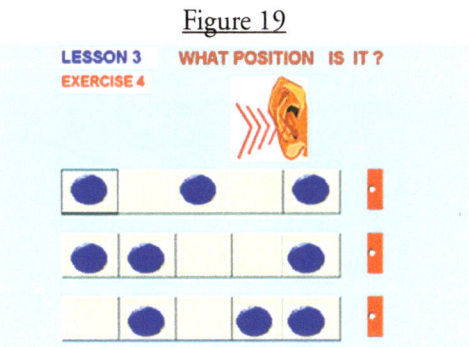

Figure 19

The answer for the audio representations is the second picture of boxes. The visual representation of the answer is indicated by a symbol in the first and second positions, followed by the third and fourth positions being left empty and finally the fifth box being filled with a symbol.

The kinesthetic representation of the answer is *clenching of the right hand* for the first and second position, followed by *clenching of the left hand* for the third and fourth positions and finally, *clenching the right hand* to represent a symbol in the fifth box.

INTRODUCTION TO POSITIONS: LESSON 20

In Figure 20 we have three combinations that contain symbols or empty squares. The audio representation of one of the pictures below is **double knock, double knock, knock, double knock, and knock.**

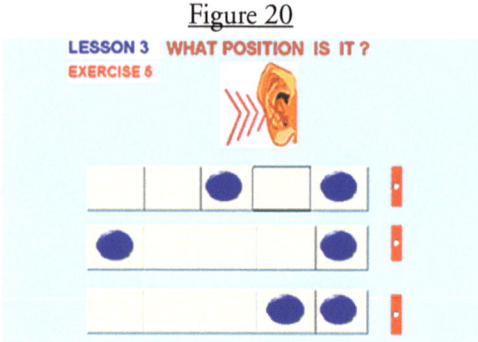

Figure 20

The answer for the audio representations is the first picture of boxes. The visual representation of the answer shows the first and second positions as empty, while the third contains a symbol. The fourth square is left empty and the fifth contains a symbol.

The kinesthetic representation of the answer is *clenching the left hand twice* for the first and second positions. The third square is represented by *clenching the right hand*, the fourth position with the *clenching of the left hand* and finally, *clenching of the right ha*nd to represent a symbol in the fifth square.

INTRODUCTION TO POSITIONS: LESSON 21

In Figure 21 we have three combinations that contain symbols or empty squares. The audio representation of one of the pictures below is **double knock, knock, double knock, knock, and knock.**

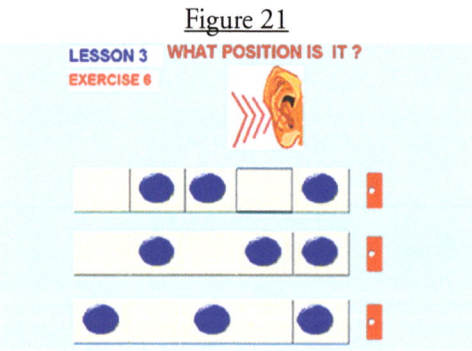

Figure 21

The answer for the audio representations is the second picture of boxes. The visual representation of the answer for the first position is an empty square followed by a symbol in the second square. The third box is empty while the fourth and fifth positions contain a symbol.

The kinesthetic representation of the answer is *clenching the left hand* for the first position, followed by the second position being represented by *clenching of the right hand*. The third square is described by *clenching of the left fist and clenching the right hand twice* represents a symbol in the fourth and fifth position.

INTRODUCTION TO POSITIONS: LESSON 22

In Figure 22 we have three combinations that contain symbols or empty squares. The audio representation of one of the pictures below is **knock, knock, double knock, double knock, and knock.**

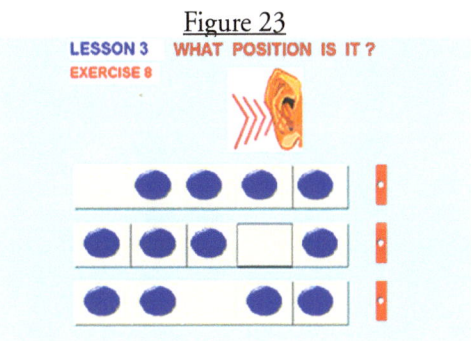

Figure 22

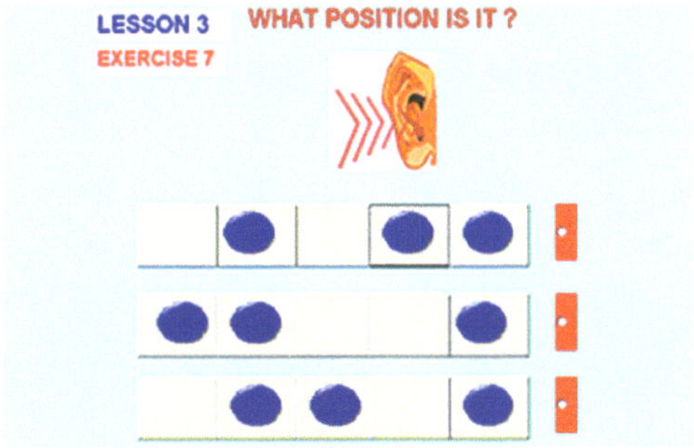

The answer for the audio representations is the second picture of the boxes. The visual description of the answer shows a symbol in the first and second position followed by empty squares in the third and fourth positions, and finally the fifth position containing a symbol.

The kinesthetic representation of the answer is *clenching of the right hand twice* for the first and second positions, followed by the third and fourth positions being represented by *clenching of the left hand twice*. Finally, *clenching of the right hand* represents a symbol in the fifth position.

INTRODUCTION TO POSITIONS: LESSON 23

In Figure 23 we have three combinations that contain symbols or empty squares. The audio representation of one of the pictures below is **knock, knock, knock, double knock, and knock.**

Figure 23

The answer for the audio descriptions is the second picture of boxes. The visual representation of the answer for the first, second and third positions contains a symbol, followed by an empty square for the fourth position while the fifth box contains a symbol.

The kinesthetic representation of the answer is *clenching of the right hand three times* for the first, second, and third position, followed by the fourth position being represented by *clenching of the left hand*. Finally *clenching of the right hand* represents a symbol in the fifth position.

INTRODUCTION TO POSITIONS: LESSON 24

In Figure 24 we have three combinations that contain symbols or empty squares. The audio representation of one of the pictures below is **double knock, double knock, double knock, knock, and knock.**

Figure 24

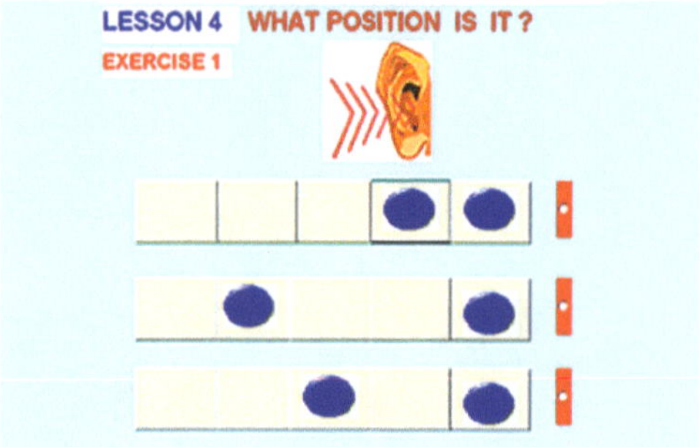

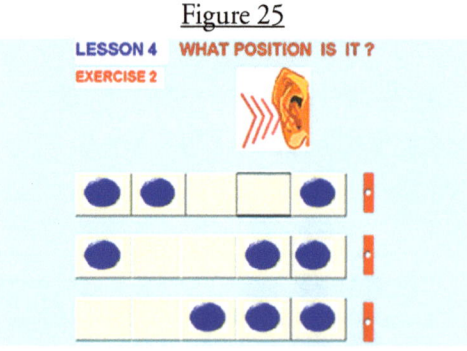

The answer for the audio representations is the first picture of boxes. The visual description of the answer is the first, second and third positions being empty while the fourth & fifth positions each contain a symbol.

The kinesthetic description of the answer is *clenching of the left hand three times* for the first, second, and third positions, followed by the fourth and fifth positions being described by *clenching of the right hand twice.*

INTRODUCTION TO POSITIONS: LESSON 25

In Figure 25 we have three combinations that contain symbols or empty squares. The audio representation of one of the pictures below is **double knock, double knock, knock, knock, and knock.**

Figure 25

The answer for the audio representation is the third picture of boxes. The visual description of the answer are empty first and second positions, while the third, fourth & fifth boxes contain a symbol.

The kinesthetic representation of the answer requires *clenching of the left hand twice* for the first and second positions, while the third, fourth and fifth positions are represented by *clenching of the right hand three times.*

INTRODUCTION TO POSITIONS: LESSON 26

In Figure 26 we have three combinations that contain symbols or empty squares. The audio representation of one of the pictures below is **double knock, knock, double knock, knock, and knock.**

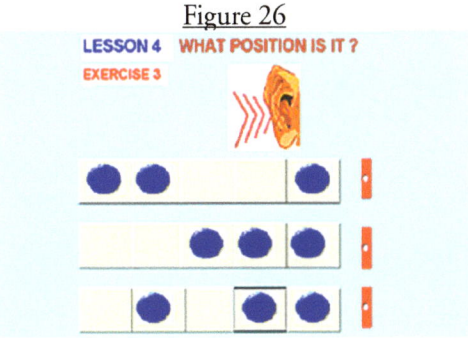

Figure 26

The answer for the audio representations is the third picture of boxes. The visual description of the answer for the first is an empty space followed by a symbol in the second position and a blank space for the third position, while the fourth & fifth positions contain symbols.

The kinesthetic representation of the answer requires *clenching of the left hand* for the first position, *clenching of the right hand* for the symbol in the second position. The third position is represented by *clenching the left hand* followed by the fourth and fifth positions being represented by *clenching the right hand twice.*

INTRODUCTION TO POSITIONS: LESSON 27

In Figure 27 we have three combinations that contain symbols or empty squares. The audio representation of one of the pictures below is **knock, double knock, knock, knock, and knock.**

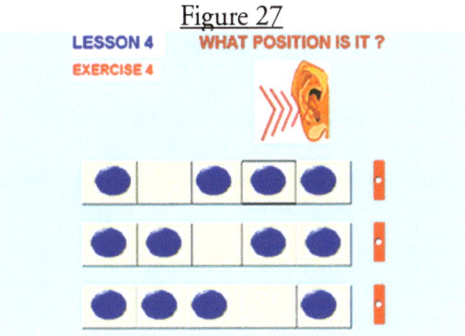

Figure 27

The answer for the audio representations is the first picture of boxes. The visual representation of the answer has a symbol in the first square followed by an empty box. The third, fourth and fifth squares each contain a symbol.
The kinesthetic representation of the answer is *clenching of the right hand* for the first position. The second position requires *clenching of the left hand* while the third, fourth and fifth are described by *clenching the right hand three times.*

INTRODUCTION TO POSITIONS: LESSON 28

In Figure 28 we have three combinations that contain symbols or empty positions. The audio representation of one of the pictures below is **double knock, double knock, knock, knock, and knock.**

<u>Figure 28</u>

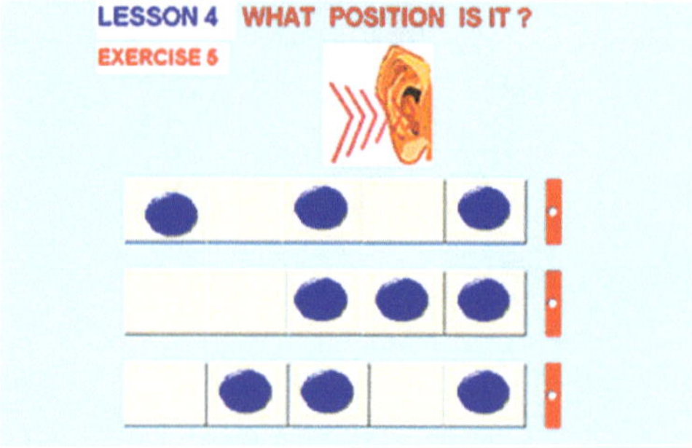

The answer for the audio representations is the second picture of boxes. In the visual representation of the answer the first and second positions are empty followed by a symbol in the third, fourth and fifth positions.

The kinesthetic representation of the answer is *clenching of the left hand twice* for the first, and second positions, while the third, fourth and fifth positions are represented by *clenching of the right hand three times*.

INTRODUCTION TO POSITIONS: LESSON 29

In Figure 29 we have three combinations that contain symbols or empty positions. The audio representation of one of the pictures below is **double knock, knock, knock, knock, and knock.**

<u>Figure 29</u>

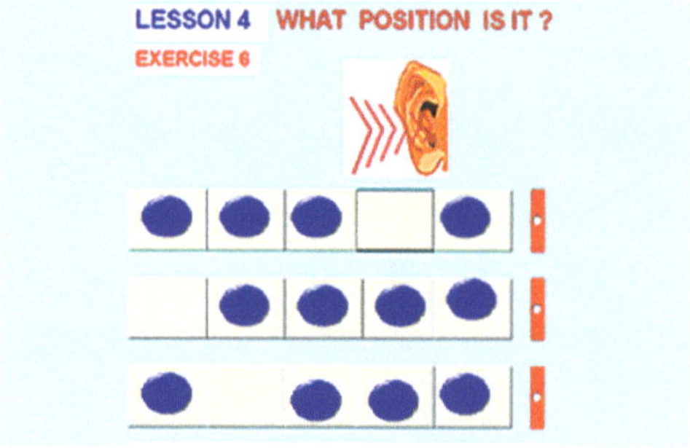

The answer for the audio representations is the second picture of boxes. The visual representation of the answer for the first position is an empty box, followed by symbols in the second, third, fourth, and fifth position.

The kinesthetic description of the answer is *clenching of the left hand* for the first position, while the second, third, fourth and fifth positions are represented by clenching of the right hand four times.

INTRODUCTION TO POSITIONS: LESSON 30

In Figure 30 we have three combinations that contain symbols or empty squares. The audio representation of one of the pictures below is **knock, knock, double knock, knock, and knock.**

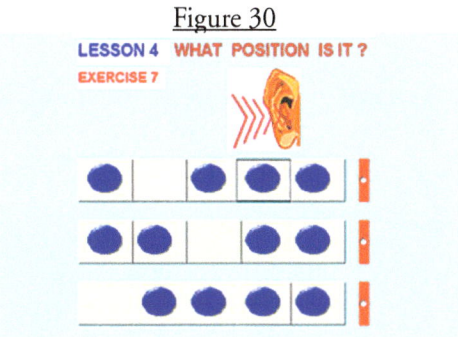

Figure 30

The answer for the audio representations is the second picture of boxes. The visual representation of the answer is a symbol in each of the first and second positions followed by an empty square in the third position. The fourth and fifth positions each contain a symbol.

The kinesthetic description of the answer is *clenching of the right hand twice* for the first and second positions, *clenching the left hand* for the third position, then *clenching of the right hand twice* for the fourth and fifth positions.

INTRODUCTION TO POSITIONS: LESSON 31

In Figure 31 we have three combinations that contain symbols or empty squares. The audio representation of one of the pictures below is **knock, knock, knock, knock, and knock.**

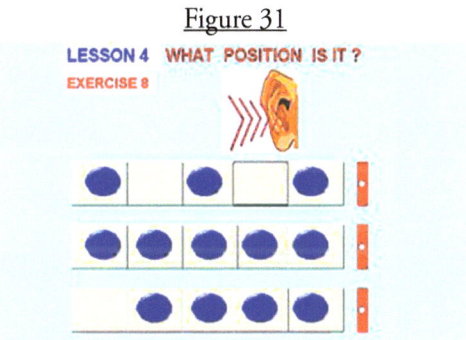

Figure 31

The answer for the audio representations is the second picture of boxes. The visual representation of the answer requires all of the squares to contain a symbol.

The kinesthetic representation of the answer is *clenching of the right hand five times* for all the positions.

INTRODUCTION TO SIGNS

INTRODUCTION TO SIGNS: LESSON ONE

There are five different signs. There is an addition sign, division sign, subtraction sign, multiplication sign, and an equal sign. Addition is represented by the sound, **tram**. Division is represented by the sound, **double click**. Subtraction is represented by the sound, **double tram**. Multiplication is represented by the sound, **blick**. The equal sign is represented by the sound, **cling**.

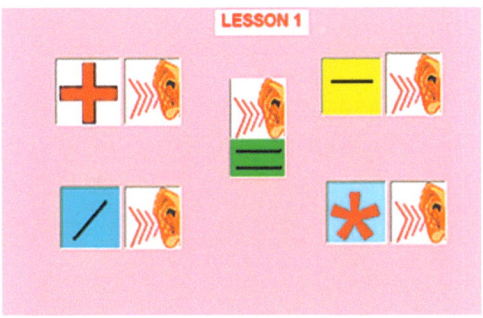

The addition sign is represented by one hand extended in front. The division sign is represented by both hands extended up. The subtraction sign is represented by both hands extended in front. The multiplication sign is represented by one hand raised up. The equal sign is represented by crossing both hands.

INTRODUCTION TO SIGNS: LESSON 1, Exercise 1

In Lesson 1 Ex. 1 there are two different signs below. The first picture is an addition sign. Addition is represented by the sound of a **tram**. The second picture is the multiplication sign. Multiplication is represented by the sound of a **blick**.

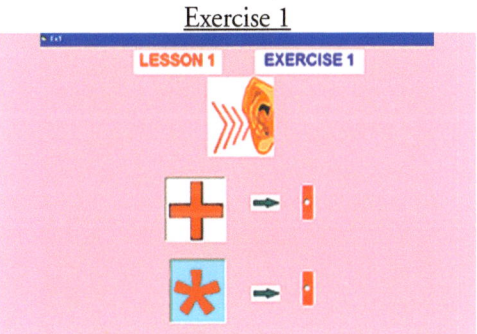

Exercise 1

The addition sign is represented by one hand extended in front. The multiplication sign is represented by one hand raised up.

INTRODUCTION TO SIGNS: LESSON 1, Exercise 2

In Lesson 1 Ex. 2 there are two different signs below. The first picture is of a subtraction sign. The subtraction sign is represented by the sound of a **double tram**. The second picture is of a division sign. The division sign is represented by the sound of a **double click**.

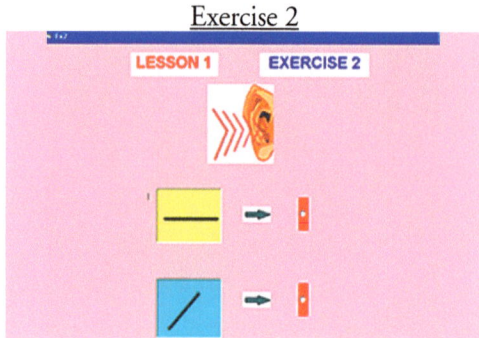

Exercise 2

The subtraction sign is represented by both hands extended in front. The division sign is represented by both hands extended up.

INTRODUCTION TO SIGNS: LESSON 1, Exercise 3

In Lesson 1 Ex. 3 there are two different signs below. The first picture is an addition sign. Addition is represented by the sound of a **tram**. The second picture is of a multiplication sign. Multiplication is represented by the sound of a **blick**.

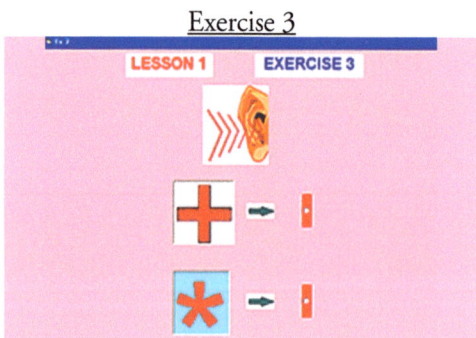

Exercise 3

The addition sign is represented by one hand extended in front. The multiplication sign is represented by one hand raised up.

INTRODUCTION TO SIGNS: LESSON 1, Exercise 4

In Lesson 1 Ex. 4 there are two different signs below. The first picture is of a multiplication sign. Multiplication is represented by the sound of a **blick**. The second picture is of a division sign. Division is represented by the sound of a **click**.

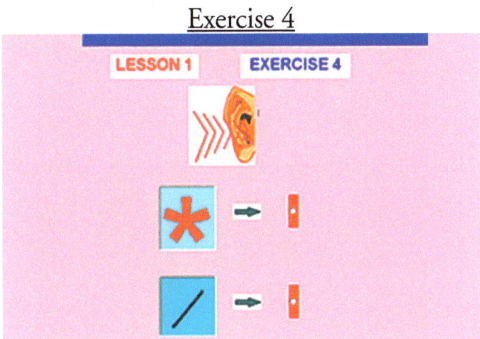

The multiplication sign is represented by one hand raised up. The division sign is represented by both hands extended up.

INTRODUCTION TO SIGNS: LESSON 1, Exercise 5

In Lesson 1 Ex. 5 there are two different signs below. The first picture is of an equal sign. The equal sign is represented by the sound of a **cling**. The second picture is of the addition sign. Addition is represented by the sound of a **tram**.

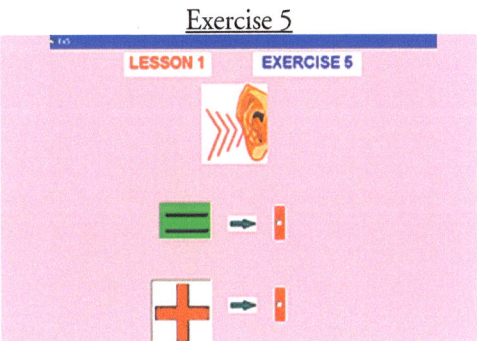

The equal sign is represented by crossing both hands. The addition sign is represented by one hand extended in front.

INTRODUCTION TO SIGNS: TRAINING, Exercise 1

In Exercise 1 Training, there are two sets of pictures below. The first picture contains an addition sign, and a multiplication sign. The sounds are represented by a **tram**, and then a **blick**. The second picture contains a division sign, and an equal sign. The sounds are represented by a **click**, and then a **cling**.

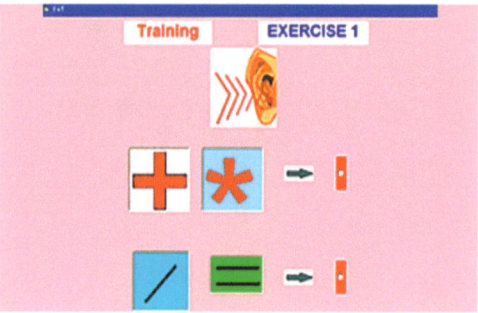

The first picture is represented by one hand extended in front, then one hand raised up. The second picture is represented by both hands extended up, then by crossing both hands.

INTRODUCTION TO SIGNS: TRAINING, Exercise 2

In Exercise 2 Training, there are two sets of pictures below. The first picture contains a division sign, and a multiplication sign. The sounds are represented by a **double click**, and then a **blick**. The second picture contains a subtraction sign, and an addition sign. The sounds are represented by a **double tram**, and then a **tram**.

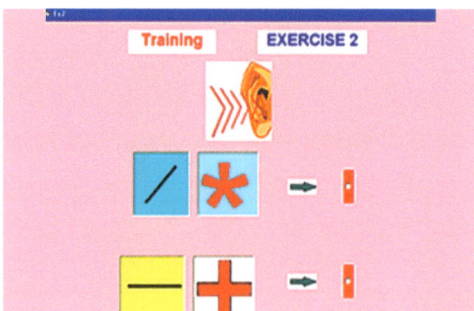

The first picture is represented by both hands extended up, then one hand raised up. The second picture is represented by both hands extended in front, then by one hand extended in front.

INTRODUCTION TO SIGNS: TRAINING, Exercise 3

In Exercise 3 Training, there are two sets of pictures below. The first picture contains a division sign, and an addition sign. The sounds are represented by a **double click**, and then a **tram**. The second picture contains a subtraction sign, and a multiplication sign. The sounds are represented by a **double tram**, and then a **blick**.

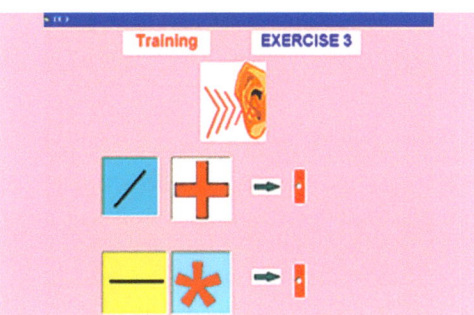

The first picture is represented by both hands extended up, then one hand extended in front. The second picture is represented by both hands extended in front, then by one hand raised up.

www.ingramcontent.com/pod-product-compliance
Lightning Source LLC
Chambersburg PA
CBHW041522220426
43669CB00002B/27